The Prescribing Pharmacist

For the full range of M&K Publishing books please visit our website:
www.mkupdate.co.uk

The Prescribing Pharmacist

Dr Barry Strickland-Hodge
Dr Mary-Claire Kennedy

The Prescribing Pharmacist

Dr Barry Strickland-Hodge and Dr Mary-Claire Kennedy (Editors)

ISBN: 978-1-910451-03-8

First published 2019

British Library Cataloguing in Publication Data
A catalogue record for this book is available from the British Library

Notice

Clinical practice and medical knowledge constantly evolve. Standard safety precautions must be followed, but, as knowledge is broadened by research, changes in practice, treatment and drug therapy may become necessary or appropriate. Readers must check the most current product information provided by the manufacturer of each drug to be administered and verify the dosages and correct administration, as well as contraindications. It is the responsibility of the practitioner, utilising the experience and knowledge of the patient, to determine dosages and the best treatment for each individual patient. Any brands mentioned in this book are as examples only and are not endorsed by the publisher. Neither the publisher nor the authors assume any liability for any injury and/or damage to persons or property arising from this publication.

To contact M&K Publishing write to:
M&K Update Ltd · The Old Bakery · St. John's Street
Keswick · Cumbria CA12 5AS
Tel: 01768 773030 · Fax: 01768 781099
publishing@mkupdate.co.uk
www.mkupdate.co.uk

Designed and typeset by Mary Blood
Printed in Scotland by Bell & Bain, Glasgow

Contents

List of contributors

Editor and contributor

Barry Strickland-Hodge BSc (Pharm), MSc, PhD, FRPharmS, FHEA
Visiting Professor of Prescribing Practice, School of Healthcare, University of Leeds

Co-editor

Mary-Claire Kennedy PhD, FHEA, MRPharmS
Module Lead for Independent and Supplementary Prescribing for Pharmacists,
Lecturer in Pharmacy Practice, School of Healthcare, University of Leeds

Contributors

Asa Auta B.Pharm, MPH, PhD
Senior Lecturer in Pharmacy Practice, University of Central Lancashire

Catherine Gill RGN, SPQ, MA, PgCert (Clinical Teaching)
Lecturer, Lead for Prescribing for Nurses and Midwives, School of Healthcare, University of Leeds;
and Lead Partner for Learning and Teaching, Caritas Group Practice

Janet Holt PhD, MPhil, BA(Hons), RGN, FHEA
Senior Lecturer, Adult Nursing, School of Healthcare, University of Leeds

Afthab Hussain BSc, PhD, PGCertHE, FHEA, FRSB
Senior Lecturer in Biomolecular Sciences, School of Life Sciences, Coventry University

Rani Khatib BPharm (Hons), PGDipClinPharm, DPharm, FRPharmS, MESC
Consultant Pharmacist in Cardiology and Cardiovascular Clinical Research
Leeds Teaching Hospitals NHS Trust

Foreword

In 1670, Jonathan Goddard, a London physician, wrote 'only doctors should prescribe' in his ongoing campaign against the encroachment of apothecaries into what he saw as his area of practice. I am an apothecary who qualified as a pharmacist in the days when Goddard's phrase still rang true. It is a joy to have been part of the development of the supplementary and then independent prescribing courses for pharmacists. Courses were accredited from 2003 and the first intake of pharmacists took place in 2004.

Changes have continued since then, with the introduction of independent prescribing courses for pharmacists, which were accredited in 2006. Initially, the range of preparations that could be prescribed by pharmacist independent prescribers was relatively limited, with no controlled drugs, though this changed again in 2012 when independent prescribers were enabled to prescribe from the whole of the British National Formulary within their limitations or scope of practice. Three drugs, when used for addiction, were excluded but this does not appear to have caused any great consternation among prescribing pharmacists to date.

When independent nurse prescribing was introduced, nurses were also unable to prescribe any controlled drug. As with pharmacists, a controlled drug was identified by adding the letters CD after the drug name, so even drugs identified with CD INV P were included in the restricted prescribing list for nurses. (It's strange to think that a nurse could buy pholcodine linctus but not prescribe it!) Unlicensed medicines were also restricted until 2012 so any mixture of two or more licensed drugs would be classed as creating an unlicensed medication and could therefore not be prescribed.

It would therefore appear that most of the barriers to a smooth transition from doctor-only prescribing to prescribing by nurses, pharmacists and other healthcare professionals, have been eradicated or at least significantly reduced. In May 2016, the General Pharmaceutical Council (GPhC) published a Prescribers Survey Report. This stated that at the beginning of November 2015 there were 3,944 annotated prescribers on the GPhC register, representing about 8% of the total number of pharmacists on the register.

This short book introduces pharmacist prescribing and begins by looking at where we are now. In 2016, the Royal Pharmaceutical Society (RPS) undertook a review of the existing competency framework and produced a more all-encompassing list of competencies to be achieved by all potential and existing prescribers, including medics, dentists, nurses and pharmacists. This list should form a major part of the work-based learning element of any prescribing course. The list of competencies is reproduced as the appendix in this book with permission of the RPS.

The body of the book considers more detailed prescribing issues, such as consultation, patient clinical assessment, working in teams, understanding cultural and religious issues and ethics. In Chapter 2, influences on the new prescriber in particular are considered. There will always be influences and attempts to make any prescriber consider new products. Medicines optimisation is another very important aspect of prescribing and for this the RPS good practice guidance is referred to in detail in Chapter 4. The book then looks at specialist patient groups, such as the elderly, the very young, pregnant women and breast-feeding women, and finally moves on to particular medicines requiring special care when prescribing.

This book is intended for any pharmacist thinking of (or interested in) the idea of pharmacist independent prescribing, those on pharmacy courses and those who are already qualified as pharmacists, who may use it as a reminder of important points covered on their course.

Barry Strickland-Hodge, *Pharmacist, Apothecary and Visiting Professor of Prescribing Practice at the University of Leeds, 2019*

References

Goddard, J.A. (1670). Discourse, setting forth the unhappy condition of the practice of physic in London. *Royal Society* VIII: 442–55 (Available at the Leeds Subscription Library).

General Pharmaceutical Council (GPhC) (2016). *Prescribers Survey Report*. https://www.pharmacyregulation.org/sites/default/files/gphc_prescribers_survey_report.pdf (last accessed 11.5.2019).

List of abbreviations

ABPM	ambulatory bp monitoring
ACEI	angiotensin converting enzyme inhibitors
APTT	activated partial thromboplastin time
AVPU	Alert, Voice, Pain, Unresponsive
BHS	British Hypertension Society
BMA	British Medical Association
BNF	British National Formulary
BNF-C	BNF for Children
BP	blood pressure
BPM	beats per minute
CAS	Central Alerting System
CCG	Clinical Commissioning Group
CD INV P	Controlled drug exempt from all requirements other than the need to retain invoices for two years
CKS	Clinical Knowledge Summary
CMDh	Coordination Group for Mutual Recognition and Decentralised Procedures-human
CMP	clinical management plan
CNS	central nervous system
COPD	chronic obstructive pulmonary disease
CPD	continuing professional development
DH	drug history
DMARD	disease-modifying anti-rheumatic drug
DN	District Nurse
DOAC	direct oral anticoagulant
dTT	dilute thrombin time
EAM	external auditory meatus
ECG	electrocardiogram
eGFR	estimated glomerular filtration rate
EHC	emergency hormonal contraception
EWTD	European Working Time Directive
FH	family history
GI	gastrointestinal
GPhC	General Pharmaceutical Council
HBPM	home blood pressure monitoring
HPC	history of presenting complaint
HRT	hormone replacement therapy
HV	Health Visitor
ICE	Ideas, Concerns and Expectations
INR	international normalised ratio

IRET	infrared in-ear thermometer
LFT	liver function test
LMWH	low molecular weight heparins
MDRD	modification of diet in renal disease
MHRA	Medicines and Healthcare products Regulatory Agency
NEWS	National Early Warning Score
NHS	National Health Service
NICE	National Institute for Health and Care Excellence
NMP	non-medical prescribing
NPSA	National Patient Safety Agency
NRLS	National Reporting and Learning System
NSAID	non-steroidal anti-inflammatory drug
OTC	over the counter
PC	presenting complaint
PDA	patient decision aid
PGD	Patient Group Direction
PIL	patient information leaflet
PLB	pursed lipped breathing
PMH	past medical history
PPI	proton pump inhibitor
QS120	Quality Standard for Medicines Optimisation
RCP	Royal College of Physicians
RI	renal impairment
RNIB	Royal National Institute of Blind People
ROS	Review of Systems
RPS	Royal Pharmaceutical Society
SBAR	Situation, Background, Assessment, Recommendation
SH	social history
SIGN	Scottish Intercollegiate Guidelines Network
SmPC	Summary of Product Characteristics
SPS	Specialist Pharmacy Service
SSRI	selective serotonin reuptake inhibitor
TAT	temporal artery thermometer
THR	traditional herbal registration
UKMi	UK Medicines Information
UKTIS	UK Teratology Information Service
WHO	World Health Organisation

1

An introduction to pharmacist prescribing

Asa Auta and Barry Strickland-Hodge

Chapter overview

In the UK and a number of other countries, many healthcare professionals, including nurses, pharmacists, optometrists, radiographers and physiotherapists, are authorised to prescribe medicines (Weeks *et al.* 2016). This chapter introduces the concept of pharmacist prescribing in the UK and briefly considers how pharmacist prescribing has been accepted and developed in other countries. The laws that govern pharmacist prescribing are considered and the Department of Health objectives for independent prescribing are described.

Introduction

In November 2015, the General Pharmaceutical Council commissioned a survey of all pharmacist prescribers on the GPhC register (GPhC 2016). At that time, the number of pharmacist prescribers was found to be almost 4000 or 8 % of the membership. Most pharmacists undertook prescribing in hospital (46 %), with 29 % in general practice and only 8 % in community pharmacy. Other areas identified were primary care organisations, care homes and prisons. The survey identified the main area of concern among prescribing pharmacists as a lack of diagnostic skills in many clinical areas. For this reason, the majority of pharmacists were prescribing only after diagnosis by another healthcare professional. Two other areas of concern were the lack of access to patients' medical records in the community and the need for a second pharmacist to provide a clinical check. Even if pharmacists intended to act only after diagnosis (adopting a collaborative approach), they still needed to have an understanding of the patient's condition and likely prognosis.

It is probably thanks to the Cumberlege report in 1986 that pharmacists gained prescribing rights in the UK as soon as they did. This report emphasised the time wasted by district nurses (DNs) and health visitors (HVs) waiting to have prescriptions signed by GPs. The initial formulary offered to DNs and HVs was short and restrictive but still enabled this group of community nurses to improve their service to patients. Once it had been demonstrated that prescribing by DNs and

HVs was safe and relevant, a broader range of nurses were included as potential prescribers and more potent medications were added to their formulary.

Although few countries have actively embraced pharmacist independent prescribing, hospital pharmacists in a number of countries have been involved in prescribing medicines under local arrangements with doctors in emergency situations (Doloresco & Vermeulen 2009). In Ghana, Tanzania, Anguilla and Argentina, for example, designated pharmacists are allowed to prescribe narcotic analgesics to cancer patients in emergency situations (Cleary & De Lima 2013). A review of the literature in 2011 showed that nurses have been authorised to prescribe in 22 countries (Bhanbhro *et al.* 2011) and in rural areas prescribing rights for nurses should be seen as essential. Definitions of what could be prescribed differ. Some countries restrict prescribing to a formulary, others to collaborations with medical practitioners only. In this latter instance the descriptive term is usually 'collaborative prescribing' (Weeks *et al.* 2016).

United Kingdom

In the United Kingdom (UK), the *Crown Report* (Department of Health 1999) used the Medicines Act (1968) definition of NHS prescribing:

> To prescribe within the National Health Service, is 'to order in writing the supply of a prescription only medicine for a named patient'. However, it was and is commonly used in the UK to authorise, by means of an NHS prescription, the supply of any medicine, at public expense.

Prescribing is separate from supply and administration. Supply was defined in the *Crown Report* as 'to provide a medicine directly to a patient or carer for administration'; and to administer is 'to give a medicine either by introduction into the body, whether by direct contact with the body or not (e.g. orally or by injection), or by external application (e.g. application of an impregnated dressing).'

Historically, prescribing had been the preserve of doctors. With the publication of the Medicines Act in 1968, prescribing was left to doctors and dentists. When the National Health Service (NHS) was developed in the UK in 1948, there were few potent drugs available to the prescriber, other than narcotics and some antibiotics. The first national formulary after 1948 contained about 400 medicines, many of which were to be compounded by the pharmacist. In 1968, when the Medicines Act was published, the number of potent medicines had increased significantly and included such drugs as hypnotics, antidepressants and antipsychotics. Pharmacy became a degree-only profession after 1967 (changing from part-degree, part-apprenticeship, perhaps in anticipation of the explosion of pharmaceuticals that followed in the 1960s, '70s and '80s).

The current British National Formulary (BNF) contains monographs for about 6,000 medicines, including different doses, dosage forms and different generic names. Prescribers must continue to keep up to date with the developing evidence when deciding upon a particular treatment for each patient. With the introduction of non-medical prescribing (NMP) – a term which now seems inappropriate as all UK prescribers are to use the same competency framework for prescribing – prescribing has been added to the remit of many additional healthcare professionals. In August 2009, the European Working Time Directive (EWTD) was fully incorporated into UK legislation. The EWTD limited workers to a maximum 48-hour week, averaged over a six-month period. The British Medical Association (BMA) reported that for junior doctors this meant that working hours were reduced from an average of 56 per week to 48, calculated over a period of 26 weeks (BMA 2016). With an ageing population living longer and potentially requiring more medicines to be prescribed, and with doctors working fewer hours, the need for more prescribers was obvious.

The two reports from Dr June Crown relating to the supply and administration of medicines were published at the end of the 1990s. Whereas the first *Crown Report* mainly reviewed the supply of medicines, it paved the way for Patient Group Directions (PGDs) among other things and strengthened and broadened the way drugs were offered to patients following consultation (Department of Health 1998).

It was the second and final *Crown Report*, published in 1999, that discussed the idea of prescribers other than doctors and dentists being given more extensive prescribing rights (Department of Health 1999). Nurses had already increased their prescribing capability with the extended formulary following additional training. Legislative change (Health and Social Care Act 2001), following the recommendations of the Crown reports, enabled nurses and pharmacists to prescribe first as supplementary prescribers then as independent prescribers (Department of Health 1998, Department of Health 1999, Cooper *et al.* 2008).

The final *Crown Report* suggested two forms of prescribing for other healthcare professionals. The first was supplementary prescribing (initially called dependent prescribing) which was introduced in 2003; and the second was independent prescribing, introduced in 2006 (Tonna *et al.* 2008). Supplementary prescribing was less controversial, as it was like other countries' collaborative prescribing in which a doctor or dentist was still required to have overall patient control. The Department of Health (2005, p. 8) definition of supplementary prescribing indicates this. It is:

> A voluntary partnership between an independent prescriber (a doctor or dentist) and a supplementary prescriber to implement an agreed patient-specific clinical management plan (CMP) with the agreement of the patient.

In the independent prescribing model (Department of Health, 2006 p.2), this was expanded to give the new independent prescriber autonomy over prescribing decisions. In this system, the prescriber is:

> ...responsible and accountable for the assessment of patients with undiagnosed or diagnosed conditions and for decisions about the clinical management required, including prescribing.

In this independent prescribing model, pharmacists took sole responsibility for every prescribing decision made, even though they may have worked in collaboration with other members of the healthcare team (Nissen 2011).

The UK Health and Social Care Act (2001) listed many other potential healthcare professionals who could, following additional training, be qualified to prescribe: some only as supplementary prescribers still requiring a doctor or dentist to make the initial diagnosis and commence treatment; others as independent but with a limited formulary. Nurses and pharmacists in the UK now have the whole BNF from which to prescribe, with the exception of three controlled drugs when used for addiction.

The Department of Health objectives for independent prescribing

In 2006, the Department of Health published objectives for the implementation of independent prescribing by those other than doctors. The aims were to:

- Improve patient care without compromising patient safety
- Make it easier for patients to get the medicines they need
- Increase patient choice in accessing medicines
- Make better use of the skills of health professionals
- Contribute to the introduction of more flexible team working across the NHS.

Requirements for independent prescribing pharmacists

The GPhC is the statutory regulator for the pharmacy profession in Great Britain. Universities wishing to offer independent prescribing courses for pharmacists must be accredited by the GPhC. The Nursing and Midwifery Council (NMC) and GPhC approved a draft curriculum and set of learning outcomes which all courses must use when developing prescribing programmes.

Accreditation ensures that universities offering such courses have the right level of support both within the university and from the staff leading and teaching on the courses. Re-accreditation takes place every three years and must meet strict criteria laid down by the GPhC. Students undertaking the prescribing course for pharmacists can be assured that the courses meet the expectation of the profession and will equip pharmacists with the basic skills required to prescribe within their level of expertise.

To qualify as a pharmacist independent prescriber, a pharmacist must currently have at least two years' post-registration experience in a patient-orientated environment, undergo study at university level equivalent to 26 days of full-time education and also undertake at least a 12-day period of learning in practice with a designated medical practitioner (Stewart et al. 2012). With the development of the new MPharm qualification in the UK incorporating, as it does, a more clinical patient- orientated approach, the requirement to undertake two years' post-registration experience may change. Likewise, qualified and trained existing pharmacist independent prescribers may become designated prescribing practitioners.

Independent pharmacist prescribers are able to initiate treatment and prescribe medicines for any condition within their clinical competence, with the exception of cocaine, dipipanone and diamorphine for treating addiction (Statutory Instrument 2012). However, in practice, many pharmacist prescribers restrict their prescribing to one specialised clinical area (Lloyd et al. 2010). Prescribing by pharmacists in the UK has been reported in many clinical areas, including infection control, pain management, hypertension, anticoagulation, diabetes, mental health and oncology. (Phelps et al. 2014).

A competency framework for prescribing

A competency framework is a collection of competencies believed to be central to the effective performance of a particular activity. Development of competencies should help individuals to continually improve their performance and to work more effectively (Whiddett & Hollyforde 1999).

Competency frameworks are used in many areas, including medicine. The competencies describe the underpinning knowledge, skills and behaviours of practitioners which must be acquired in order for the individual to be assessed as competent. A single set of competencies has been developed to cover all prescribing practitioners. These competencies must be achieved and maintained to demonstrate safe and effective prescribing competence.

All prescribing is underpinned by legislation and regulatory standards. Accordingly, all pharmacist prescribers in Great Britain must record their qualification with the General Pharmaceutical Council (GPhC). They also have a responsibility to keep their knowledge and skills up to date, to ensure that they are able to prescribe competently and safely.

Continuing professional development (CPD) for pharmacists, who are also prescribers, should include CPD related to their prescribing.

The UK Competency Framework for All Prescribers

In the UK, profession-specific prescribing competency frameworks were developed by the National Prescribing Centre (NPC), starting with the outline framework for nurse prescribers in 2001. This first edition was reviewed and updated in 2003. The first set of competencies specifically for pharmacists was also published in 2003, when pharmacist supplementary prescribing was first introduced. To support all prescribers to prescribe effectively, a single prescribing competency framework was published in 2012. This was widely used as part of prescribing course design and accreditation. References to each of these competency frameworks can be found in the Royal Pharmaceutical Society (RPS) Prescribing Framework Report (RPS 2016).

The 2012 framework was due for review in 2014. The RPS was approached to manage the update of the framework on behalf of all the prescribing professions in the UK. To ensure that the framework was applicable across the whole of the UK, representatives of the Chief Pharmaceutical Officers of England, Scotland, Wales and Northern Ireland, as well as Health Education England, NHS Education for Scotland and NICE, were represented on a project board (RPS 2016).

The Competency Framework for All Prescribers sets out what good prescribing looks like. There are ten competencies split into two domains: Consultation and Prescribing. Within each of the ten competency dimensions, there are statements describing the skills or outcomes competent prescribers should be able to demonstrate (see Appendix).

The prescribing framework is applicable to any prescriber, regardless of their professional background. It may therefore need contextualising to reflect different specialties and prescribing expertise.

The basic framework covers all aspects of prescribing, from having up-to-date clinical knowledge to making or reviewing a diagnosis, sharing decisions, being safe, being professional, understanding the healthcare system, knowing how to get additional information, working with others, reflecting on practice and undertaking CPD. They offer a guide to what all prescribers should know and should be the basis for any workplace assessment for pharmacists undertaking prescribing programmes.

Throughout this short book, we refer to this 2016 competency framework and the competencies are reproduced with permission from the RPS as the appendix.

Summary

This chapter has introduced the concept of pharmacist prescribing in the UK and briefly considered how pharmacist prescribing has developed in other countries. It looked briefly at the laws that govern pharmacist independent prescribing and the Department of Health objectives for introducing it. Finally, the chapter considered prescribing competencies and, in particular, the UK Competency Framework for All Prescribers.

References

Bhanbhro, S., Drennan, V.M. *et al.* (2011). Assessing the contribution of prescribing in primary care by nurses and professionals allied to medicine: a systematic review of literature. *BMC Health Services Research*. **11**, 330.

British Medical Association (BMA) (2016). *European Working Time Directive: Junior doctors FAQ*. https://www.bma.org.uk/advice/employment/working-hours/ewtd (last accessed 14.5.2019).

Canadian Pharmacists Association (CPhA) (2011). *CPhA Position Statement on Pharmacist Prescribing*. http://www.pharmacists.ca/cpha-ca/assets/File/cpha-on-the-issues/PPPharmacistPrescribing.pdf (last accessed 14.5.2019).

Cleary, J. & De Lima, L. (2013). Formulary availability and regulatory barriers to accessibility of opioids for cancer pain in Latin America and the Caribbean: a report from the Global Opioid Policy Initiative (GOPI). *Annals of Oncology*. **24**, xi41–xi50.

Cockburn, J. & Pit, S. (1997). Prescribing behaviour in clinical practice: patients' expectations and doctors' perceptions of patients' expectations – a questionnaire study. *British Medical Journal*. **315**, 520.

Cooper, R., Guillaume, L. *et al.* (2008). Nonmedical prescribing in the United Kingdom: developments and stakeholder interests. *The Journal of Ambulatory Care Management*. **31**, 244–52.

Department of Health (1998). *Review of prescribing, supply and administration of medicines: a report on the supply and administration of medicines under group protocols*. https://webarchive.nationalarchives.gov.uk/20030731075216/http://www.doh.gov.uk:80/protocol.htm (last accessed 14.5.2019).

Department of Health (1999). *Review of prescribing, supply and administration of medicines. Final*. https://www.publichealth.hscni.net/sites/default/files/directorates/files/Review%20of%20prescribing,%20supply%20and%20administration%20of%20medicines.pdf (last accessed 14.5.2019).

Department of Health (2005). *Supplementary prescribing by nurses, pharmacists, chiropodists/podiatrists, physiotherapists and radiographers within the NHS in England: a guide for implementation*. https://webarchive.nationalarchives.gov.uk/20070306020119/http://www.dh.gov.uk/assetRoot/04/11/00/33/04110033.pdf (last accessed 14.5.2019).

Department of Health (2006). *Improving patients' access to medicines: a guide to implementing nurse and pharmacist independent prescribing within the NHS in England*. https://webarchive.nationalarchives.gov.uk/20130105033522/http://www.dh.gov.uk/prod_consum_dh/groups/dh_digitalassets/@dh/@en/documents/digitalasset/dh_4133747.pdf (last accessed 14.5.2019).

Doloresco, F. & Vermeulen, L.C. (2009). Global survey of hospital pharmacy practice. *American Journal of Health-System Pharmacy*. **66**, s13–s19.

General Pharmaceutical Council (GPhC) (2016). *Prescribers Survey Report*. https://www.pharmacyregulation.org/sites/default/files/gphc_prescribers_survey_report.pdf (last accessed 14.5.2019).

Health and Social Care Act (2001). Section 63. London. https://www.legislation.gov.uk/ukpga/2001/15/section/63 (last accessed 14.5.2019).

Lloyd, F., Parsons, C. *et al.* (2010). 'It's showed me the skills that he has': pharmacists' and mentors' views on pharmacist supplementary prescribing. *International Journal of Pharmacy Practice*. **18**, 29–36.

Mulholland, P. (2012). Pharmacist prescribing in neonatal intensive care units in the UK. *Archives of Disease in Childhood*. 98:e 1

Nissen, L. (2011). Pharmacist prescribing: what are the next steps? *American Journal of Health-System Pharmacy*. **68**, 2357–61.

PCNZ (2011). *Accreditation Standards for the Prescribed Qualification: Pharmacist Prescriber Scope of Practice*. http://www.pharmacycouncil.org.nz/New-Zealand-Registered-Pharmacists/Interns-Pharmacists-and-Pharmacist-Prescribers/Pharmacist-Prescribers (last accessed 14.5.2019).

Phelps, A., Agur, M., *et al.* (2014). *GPhC Registrant survey 2013*. London: NatCen Social Research.

Royal Pharmaceutical Society (RPS) (2016). *A Competency Framework for All Prescribers*. Royal Pharmaceutical Society, London. https://www.rpharms.com/Portals/0/RPS%20document%20library/Open%20access/Professional%20standards/Prescribing%20competency%20framework/prescribing-competency-framework.pdf (last accessed 14.5.2019).

Statutory Instrument (2012). *The Misuse of Drugs* (Amendment No.2) (England, Wales and Scotland) Regulations. Statutory Instrument No. 973. Stationery Office http://www.legislation.gov.uk/uksi/2012/973/made (last accessed 14.5.2019).

Stewart, D., Maclure, K. *et al.* (2012). Educating nonmedical prescribers. *British Journal of Clinical Pharmacology.* **74**, 662–67.

Tonna, A.P., Stewart, D. *et al.* (2008). An international overview of some pharmacist prescribing models. *Journal of the Malta College of Pharmacy Practice.* Issue 14, Summer, 20–26.

Weeks, G., George, J. *et al.* 2016. Non-medical prescribing versus medical prescribing for acute and chronic disease management in primary and secondary care. *Cochrane Database of Systematic Reviews.* 22, 11. CD011227.

Whiddett, S. & Hollyforde, S. (1999). *The Competencies Handbook*. Chartered Institute of Personnel & Development.

2

The consultation, diagnostic process, diagnosis and influences on prescribing

Catherine Gill and Barry Strickland-Hodge

Chapter overview

In order to recognise the patient as a 'partner' in the consultation, the practitioner must create an environment that places the patient at the centre. The processes in the consultation and eventual diagnosis and follow-up correspond to many of the competencies within the Competency Framework for all Prescribers (see Appendix). When it comes to prescribing, it needs to be borne in mind that decisions can often be influenced by outside sources and agencies. This chapter provides an overview of the skills needed to achieve the competencies effectively.

The following competencies are discussed in this chapter:

1. Assess the patient
2. Consider the options
3. Reach a shared decision
4. Provide information
5. Monitor and review

As well as part of all the Competencies related to Governance 7–10 (RPS 2016; see Appendix).

To prescribe safely and effectively, prescribers need a good knowledge of a specialist area of practice, including drug choices available. The prescribing decision should firstly be based on a thorough clinical assessment of the patient and gathering all necessary information through a medical and medication history. Secondly, all prescribers need an ability to listen and assimilate what they are hearing and seeing and an ability to communicate their conclusions and rationale to the patient or their carer/representative in a manner that can be easily understood. This may mean adjusting the communication style to suit or match the patient. Ensuring that the consultation is a partnership is key – the patient, as will be shown, has the last word.

Prescriptions may be issued for a number of reasons, other than a clearly defined clinical need. For instance, the prescription may cover a lack of clarity in the patient's condition while waiting for further results, or it could be considered a justifiable empirical treatment based on experience. At worst, the prescription could be used to end the consultation.

Introduction

It can be argued that the consultation, including observing signs and symptoms, is the most important aspect of prescribing. Get this wrong and the eventual choice of medication and/or choice of treatment will be adversely affected. Effective communication has an enormous impact on the quality of patient care. Indeed, the way in which healthcare practitioners communicate with patients may be as important as the actual information being delivered (McEwen & Harris 2010). Shared decision-making incorporates communication between healthcare practitioners, patients and carers; and this communication involves complex reasoning and processing skills. If these skills are well developed, the patient is more likely to adhere to any agreed plan and is also therefore more likely to benefit from complying with the recommended treatment. This is covered by Competency 3, statement 3.1: 'works with the patient/carers in partnership to make informed choices agreeing a plan that respects patient preferences including their right to refuse or limit treatment' (RPS 2016; see Appendix).

One of the most important factors in establishing a patient-centred consultation is the practitioner's interpersonal skills. These include projecting a caring and interested attitude, correctly interpreting the patient's agenda and discussing options in a clear and concise way. Listening for verbal cues, as well as monitoring and understanding the patient's body language, will aid the practitioner in making an initial diagnosis. Simply put, if the correct diagnosis is made, the patient is likely to receive the correct treatment, which may or may not involve prescribing medication.

If the outcome of the consultation is a prescription, remember that all medicines have side effects. If any potential side effects are discussed with the patient, and they know what to expect, they can make an informed decision about the medicines they are being asked to take. By gathering as much information as possible from the patient, including the patient's beliefs about medicine taking, their expectations and their possible concerns, the practitioner will be able to support and guide patients regarding any suggested treatment. Research shows that this type of inclusive approach usually leads to better outcomes for patients, while the 'paternalistic' (or clinician-centric) style often results in poorer adherence to a medical regimen (Jagosh et al. 2011, Lado et al. 2008, Mustafa et al. 2014).

Pharmacists learn to analyse information, whether for chemical analysis or as a basis for scientific papers. The consultation can be seen as another form of analysis, following the process of information-gathering and interpretation. Thorough information-gathering and analysis influence the precision of diagnosis and therefore treatment. Patients often believe the opposite, weighting physical examination and laboratory or imaging tests as the most important. A rapport is needed with each patient to ensure they feel comfortable discussing their problems. The outcome of the consultation depends on the practitioner's clinical knowledge and skills, experience and interviewing technique. The behaviour of the practitioner, and their attitude towards the patient, are as important as what is said. The ultimate aim is to be able to undertake high-level reasoning, incorporating physical examination if appropriate, while remaining caring.

Models of consultation

Models of consultation offer a supportive framework within which the practitioner can work. A model of consultation is not meant to be a set of rigid rules but it can offer a way forward to ensure a satisfactory outcome for both prescriber and patient. The goal of a prescriber is to obtain as much information from the patient as time allows. It is useful to develop an inventory of staple phrases for the opening greeting. Open questions allow probing, while closed questions will assist in efficient analysis (Gill & Murphy 2014). Some models of consultation concentrate on tasks and skills, while others focus more on process and outcome. Many concentrate on the relationship between the prescriber and the patient and others are more person-centred. The Enhanced Calgary–Cambridge approach (Kurtz et al. 2003) is the most commonly taught and used model in the UK (Gillard & Benson et al. 2009). It is suitable for both primary care and secondary care settings, although it was initially written for family doctors and may need to be adapted to suit different settings and clinical fields. It can be found on the gp-training.net website. The full link is shown in the references.

There is an obvious power imbalance between patient and prescriber (McEwen & Harris 2010). Understanding and addressing this issue can help the flow of information between the patient and the prescriber. It may also help the practitioner interpret what the patient is trying to communicate (Birks & Watt 2007). Developing a rapport with the patient early on in the consultation will yield dividends in tackling some of the power imbalance, and will put both the prescriber and the patient on an equal footing.

Developing a rapport

The patient needs to feel confident that the prescriber knows what they are doing and that they are the right person to deal with their problem. The patient may begin their assessment of the prescriber before the consultation even begins. For example, conventional notions of what a pharmacist does may influence their expectations either negatively or positively. The first encounter with a patient in an advanced role (such as that of a prescribing pharmacist) is therefore potentially fraught with dissonance.

Greetings and introductions

A registered pharmacist is expected to project a professional and respectful persona; yet this advanced role requires these qualities to be equally balanced with a caring approach. There are no second chances to make a first impression. Making the patient feel comfortable and welcome from the outset may offset any stereotypical ideas about pharmacists. This may be partly achieved by the way the patient is greeted. For example, offering a handshake may be one approach or, if in a consulting room, standing up when the patient comes in. Sometimes simply smiling and gesturing towards a seat may be all that is needed. Remember that not everyone wants to be addressed by their first name. In order to reduce the likelihood of getting off on the wrong foot, it may be wise to start by assuming that all patients want to be known by their surname and title.

Positioning and active listening

Following greeting and introduction, the prescriber should ensure that there are no physical barriers between them and the patient. In a hospital setting, it's best to stand at the side of the bed, not at the end. If in a consulting room, ensure the chairs are positioned without a desk between prescriber and patient (Jagosh *et al.* 2011). In the community, pharmacists are always on the front line and deal with patients all day but how often is there a counter between them and the patient? Most hospital pharmacists will also see patients – but not all will deal with them directly. There is a big difference between being a good pharmacist or clinical pharmacist and being a prescriber.

If the patient is returning to a clinic, the notes should be checked first to ensure there is an awareness of who the patient is and why they have re-attended. Does age and/or gender alter the way the consultation is started? Highly important at this stage is how long to give the patient to disclose their reason for attendance. Giving time after welcoming them, even though this silence may be uncomfortable, may save time later. This period of listening (known as the 'golden minute') ensures the patient feels able to give all the relevant and necessary information. The urge to interject should be controlled; the patient should be listened to without interruption. According to Moulton, this also has a psychological benefit and patients will be more likely to feel the prescriber has empathy and understands them (Moulton 2007, p. 23). This can be called the beginning of 'person-centeredness'.

Listening can be even more powerful if other observable behaviours are used in conjunction with it, thus making it into active listening. Active listening incorporates interpersonal skills such as smiling at appropriate times, making (and maintaining) eye contact and nodding, with facial expressions that indicate comprehension and interest.

Continuing the enquiry and exploration

Once the patient has finished giving their account of the problem, an initial analysis may be made, leading to a number of potential differential diagnoses. However, before testing any of these suppositions, the patient should be asked if there is anything else they would like to mention. This may not reveal anything new but it gives them a moment to consider any other potentially important points.

The likeliest diagnosis should be tested first and an attempt should be made to rule out the least likely explanation. Open questions should be asked at this stage, without any suggestion of a preferred answer. For example, if a patient presenting with a headache is asked 'Your headache doesn't wake you at night, does it?' this is a closed question, inviting a yes or no reply. It also has a negative bias. Asking 'Tell me more about the nature of your headache. When does it occur and are there any triggers?' is neutral and will produce a richer narrative. In this way, open questions direct the patient to think beyond the most noticeable aspects of the problem and confirm whether there is anything else that might be relevant to the diagnosis but might not necessarily be in the forefront of their mind.

At this stage, the most important part of the consultation needs to be considered – differential diagnoses, followed by a diagnosis. All the information gathered so far needs to be synthesised and assimilated. As part of the penultimate analysis, closed questions should be used to further reduce the differentials and firm up a 'working diagnosis'. Closed questions assist in confirming or refuting the working diagnosis, which may be further differentiated by means of investigations such as blood tests and imaging as necessary.

Summarising the information gathered so far

The final element of the information-gathering stage of the consultation is summarising (for the patient) what the practitioner believes the patient has described. If the summary isn't correct, or something has been missed, the patient will correct this. The patient should first be asked to summarise what has been discussed to ensure the information has been assimilated correctly by both parties. With practice, this becomes a natural part of the conversation, rather than an awkward addition.

Although the patient may have openly discussed their symptoms, it is important to know what, if anything, they are worried or concerned about and indeed what treatment they believe will be the likely outcome. It's important to pitch this conversation correctly. For example, a question such as 'What do you think is wrong and what do you think the treatment might be?' may convey a level of incompetence. In contrast, saying something like 'You have clearly given this a lot of thought. Is there anything you are worried this might be and have you thought about the possible treatment options?' is more likely to stimulate a frank disclosure. Exploring patients' Ideas, Concerns and Expectations (ICE) is considered to be an essential element in a patient-centred consultation and is also known to reduce assumptions on the part of the prescriber. Matthys *et al.* (2009) found an association between the presence of patient concerns and/or expectations, and less medication prescribing. The data from their study also suggested that exploring ICE components might lead to fewer new medication prescriptions.

Taking a medical history

Generations of doctors and diagnostic clinicians have been taught a system of medical interviewing known as the traditional model. This model can be traced back to post-Revolutionary France; and by 1880 it was firmly established as the only way to take a patient history. It involves following a standard formula of data collection that can be used to help solve the diagnostic puzzle (Silverman 2014, p. 459). This framework can be neatly inserted into any patient-centred approach to facilitate a logical approach to the diagnostic process.

The traditional model

- PC (Presenting Complaint) – what is the patient's current problem? Do not come to a conclusion about what is wrong without finishing the consultation process. For example, the patient may say they have a chest infection but this is not the presenting complaint.

The presenting symptom is a cough; and the cough may not be due to an infection. It may, for instance, be a side effect of medication or a presenting symptom of heart failure.

- HPC (History of Presenting Complaint) – how long has it been happening? Does anything make it better or worse? Was there anything that initiated the symptom(s)? Are there any associated symptoms?
- PMH (Past Medical History) – ask the patient to give a summary of medical problems not included in the HPC.
- DH (Drug History) – see below. An adverse drug reaction should always be considered as a possible indication of presenting symptoms.
- FH (Family History) – relevant diseases of close family members (such as diabetes, heart disease, stroke and cancer) should be noted, as should the age and cause of death if family members are deceased.
- SH (Social History) – alcohol use, smoking status, recreational drug use. It may be relevant to find out who the patient lives with (they may be cared for, or they may be a carer) or to ascertain if they are vulnerable themselves. Other pertinent social information may include occupation, exercise and normal activities of daily living.
- ROS (Review of Systems) – the common characteristic constellation of signs and symptoms and the conditions underlying them in each major body system must be known in advance. Using the above example of a cough as the PC, it may be important to review the respiratory and cardiovascular systems (Silverman 2014, p. 459).

Taking a medication history

Before any prescribing decisions can be taken, it is necessary to make a complete list of medications the patient is currently taking. Pharmacists will take a medication history, and investigate why patients are taking what they are taking. However, their motive will not be to 'police' other prescribers but to diagnose and treat.

The first question to ask (even if the patient's notes are available) is 'What medicines have you been prescribed?' Of course it helps if the patient record is available on screen or in hard copy. However, it's not only prescribed medicines from pharmacies that are important but any active medication from several other potential 'outlets' – such as supermarkets, healthfood shops, the internet and friends or neighbours.

This information needs to be obtained in a systematic reproducible way. Asking 'What are you taking currently?' is unlikely to produce complete results unless the answer is 'Nothing'. Pharmacists know that patients don't always think of products they have bought at the supermarket as medicines, and may not realise that inhalers and patches can also be medicines. Medicines in the form of suppositories, or an inhaler, could be missed, unless they are specifically asked about. Some are potent and could interact if absorbed.

Likewise, if patients have used 'alternative medicines' (such as herbal medicines), they may not realise these are relevant unless the prescriber undertakes some form of probing. Herbal remedies, for instance, may have active ingredients that could potentially interact with the patient's prescribed medicines. Drug interactions can occur between prescribed medicines but also between prescribed and 'over the counter' (OTC) medicines.

It isn't always easy to find out about herbs and their active ingredients. However, the Medicines and Healthcare products Regulatory Agency (MHRA) have a link which should help you find the summary of product characteristics (SPC) and the patient information leaflet (PIL) for those herbs that have a traditional herbal registration (THR). Details of the summary of product characteristics and patient leaflets for products registered under the THR scheme are available on: http://www.mhra.gov.uk/spc-pil/index.htm

The patient's medication record needs to be identified and checked if it's available. If this record isn't available, proceed with caution. It may be that whatever was prescribed isn't being taken for some reason. It's important to ascertain this reason in order to ensure that the same or similar medication isn't given again. Alternatively, the previously prescribed medicine may be being taken or used but not being used correctly. A simple discussion may sort out the problem. Does the patient know why they were prescribed the medicines they are taking? Asking about how they take their medicines may reveal that they have stopped or cut down, or even increased, the recommended dose. An explanation of the reason why they are taking the medicine may have been missed the first time.

Patients may only have heard that they require medication as treatment but the instructions may have been lost. The pharmacy should of course pick this up but it may still have been missed. In the hospital setting, it may be the clinical/prescribing pharmacist's role to 'clerk' the patient and this involves undertaking a medication history and ensuring a reconciliation of medicines. Some medicines will be essential and must be continued but others may be unnecessary or potentially causing problems and these should be identified.

Identifying drug allergies is essential; obviously it is vital not to give a drug or constituent to which the patient is allergic. Allergies mean different things to different people but the patient's view should be taken as correct at least at the initial stages. Allergy or hypersensitivity status can be considered again later to establish whether there is a true allergy so the necessary action can be taken.

What makes a good medication history?

It is important to have a full medication history to ensure that the prescriber:

- Understands the problem fully and where it fits in the patient's current medical picture. Could their current complaint be a worsening of an existing problem, a side effect of current medication (prescribed or non-prescribed), a drug–drug or drug–disease interaction, a result of incorrect medication usage or a consequence of the patient's lifestyle?
- Knows whether there may be any potential communication difficulties. Does the patient have hearing or learning difficulties, mental health problems or a social situation that may affect a prescribing decision for related and unrelated complaints?
- Can predict any potential problems resulting from the prescribing decision and put steps in place to minimise these. This may involve screening or follow-up tests, a follow-up appointment, or a referral to a specialist.

- Can avoid unwanted duplication of medications.
- Can accurately interpret any laboratory tests. For example, amiodarone may affect laboratory thyroid function tests, and the consumption of alcohol and other medication or the presence of infection can affect a patient's international normalised ratio (INR) if they are on warfarin.
- Tailor any patient education to fit the individual patient's needs.

Confirming details

Open questions will elicit the most accurate information even though this takes more time than closed questions. For example, it's better to ask 'Can you tell me how you are taking your bisoprolol at the moment?' rather than 'You're taking 2.5mg of bisoprolol every morning, is that right?'. Closed questions lead the patient to a certain answer. This type of question may convey to the patient what it is thought they should be doing and a number of patients may want to please the prescriber and respond by saying 'yes', even though they may be unsure about how to take the medication or even deliberately taking it incorrectly. When it comes to allergies, it is also important to check medical history details. Asking 'Do you have any allergies?' may elicit a 'no' from the patient. But if there are documented allergies on the screen, the practitioner needs to check further by saying, for instance: 'Your record shows that you're allergic to penicillin. Is this incorrect?'

It is, of course, important to be satisfied that the patient is able to give reliable, good-quality information and take into account the possibility of, for example, acute and chronic confusion, memory loss and the presence of family members/friends who may cause distractions and/or influence the answers given by the patient. Remember, cognitive confusion is not restricted to the elderly population.

Information must be gathered in a systematic reproducible way. Again, there are many different models for this (Nickless & Noble 2009). Although it is not simple to remember, the mnemonic PAKASPO CHIPES CRIB covers what is needed for a basic medication history (Gill & Murphy 2014). Each of the letters of the mnemonic is described in turn, and the way they can be used to elicit the medication history is discussed.

PAKASPO CHIPES CRIBS

PRESCRIPTION ONLY MEDICINES
Which drugs have been prescribed? List them, with the dose and frequency. The patient's record should be checked to see if they match.

ADHERENCE
The patient should be asked if they take their medicines in accordance with instructions discussed and agreed to at a previous consultation. This provides an opportunity to check whether too much or too little is being taken, and why.

KNOWLEDGE
Does the patient know what each type of medication is for? If not, this is an opportunity to explain. If the patient is unsure, they may not be taking their medication correctly.

ALLERGIES

As mentioned above, allergies are difficult. A patient may assume that a stomach upset occurring at the same time as taking a medicine is an allergy, when there could be another explanation. Nevertheless, their statement should be taken into account and accepted; its accuracy can be examined later if necessary.

SIDE EFFECTS

Has the patient noticed any side effects since starting the medication? All drugs have side effects and some may be severe enough to stop the patient taking the medicine. (For instance, many types of medication have gastro-intestinal effects.) Reassurance may be all that is needed – or an alternative prescription if the side effects are unacceptable.

PHARMACY MEDICINES

Many pharmacy medicines have potent ingredients and these need to be noted. If they are being obtained regularly, find out why this is and whether support can be offered. It might be relevant to ask here also about purchased vitamins and dietary supplements.

OVER THE COUNTER MEDICINES

Small amounts of analgesics or antihistamines may have been bought from a supermarket and these may interact with other medications or have their own side effects. Possible internet purchases should also be considered.

CREAMS, LOTIONS, GELS

Why is the patient using cream, lotion or gel? Is it for an itch possibly brought on by one of the other medicines? This may also lead into a more general discussion of skin complaints.

HERBAL

Does the herbal remedy have a traditional herbal registration (THR)? Is the patient using the herbal medicine for the same reasons they are receiving the prescription medicine? Is the herb mentioned in the *British National Formulary* (BNF)? Or the MHRA (2019) website can be consulted. Vitamins and dietary supplements should be considered if not already identified in the 'pharmacy medicines' section of the mnemonic.

INHALERS

Sometimes patients forget that inhalers are also medicines. Breathlessness may have been the reason why they were given an inhaler – is it still needed?

PATCHES

Many medicines are commonly delivered by patch and these can have unforeseen effects on the patient. For instance, side effects from nicotine replacement patches or HRT patches need to be taken into account.

EYE/EAR/NASAL DROPS

These may well be local-action but eye drops can also be absorbed and have systemic actions.

SUPPOSITORIES/PESSARIES

Finally, suppositories and pessaries should be considered. If used for local action, they may not be relevant; but if they are absorbed, their action needs to be identified.

CONTRACEPTION

If appropriate, ask about forms of contraception, including oral contraceptive pill, injectable, implant and coil.

RECREATIONAL DRUGS

There are a number of drugs that produce 'highs', as well as other illegal substances which may have an effect on other medicines prescribed or to be prescribed (enzyme inhibitors and enhancers) that should be identified. When asking about the use of these substances, it is vital to pitch the question in a relaxed manner. 'Do you take any recreational drugs?' should be asked in the same tone as the rest of the interview. If the practitioner is hesitant or embarrassed, there is a risk the patient may not be honest.

INTERNET PURCHASED DRUGS

People are increasingly buying medication online and this needs to be discussed. This could be asked in the 'pharmacy medicines' or the 'OTC' sections of the mnemonic. Herbals, vitamins and dietary supplements are frequently advertised as 'natural' on the internet so patients may not think they need to be mentioned. If this is not picked up, in the 'herbal' or 'OTC' sections of the mnemonic, it could be picked up here.

BORROWED MEDICATION

A patient's friend, relative or colleague may have had a positive effect from a particular medication and recommended it for this patient's problem. The question 'Do you ever take anyone else's medication?' may guide the patient to volunteer the information at this point.

Other substances that can have an effect on prescribed medication include tobacco and alcohol (which are enzyme inhibitors and enhancers). This should have been picked up in the social section of the medical history. Could any of these social substances have an interaction with a prescribed drug and potentially be the cause of the patient's visit today?

Medicine-taking behaviour: Compliance, adherence and concordance

Competency 1 in the Competency Framework is 'Assess the patient'. Statement 7 says 'reviews adherence to and effectiveness of current medicines' (RPS 2016; see Appendix). The terms compliance, adherence and concordance are well known. They are considered very superficially here, identifying the main differences and how understanding them can help support the patient. A word like 'compliance' is paternalistic and clinician-centric – in other words, the antithesis of patient-centred practice. 'Adherence' more accurately describes whether or not a patient is taking their medicines in accordance with an agreed plan or indeed prescriber instructions. Non-adherence may be a simple case of not realising how important it is to continue; or it may occur because of side effects or for a number of other reasons – for instance, the prescriber may have issued instructions without first enquiring if a particular medication was what the patient was expecting or wanting. Non-adherence is a known multi-factorial issue and a much-researched subject. Adherence and non-adherence are discussed in more detail in Chapter 4 (Patient partnership and prescribing).

Analysing and evaluating the information

It is estimated that 80% of a patient's assessment takes place during the history-taking process, including observation. Observation begins as soon as the patient presents at the surgery or hospital. Important information can be gathered from the patient's physical appearance, such as gait, facial expression, skin colouration, etc. A number of disorders present with recognisable outward signs – for example, endocrine conditions can present with signs and symptoms such as hair thinning, sweating and so on. Linking these observations to the history the patient is relaying will help the practitioner arrive at a final diagnosis.

Diagnostic competence is governed by knowledge and understanding of the patient's problem. The practitioner also needs specific knowledge of the disease differentials likely to have caused the problem and an understanding of when the working diagnosis needs to be tested further with a physical examination and near-patient tests. Near-patient tests are tests that give speedy results such as urinalysis, blood glucose and electrocardiogram. Always remember to check both urinalysis and blood glucose in a patient who is presenting with confusion.

The GPhC are clear that pharmacist prescribers should be able to undertake an appropriate clinical physical examination commensurate with the advanced role of a prescriber. In Competency 1 ('Assess the patient'), Statement 2 is 'undertakes an appropriate clinical assessment'. Chapter 3 goes into detail about some red flags and basic clinical assessment.

The main objective is to exclude the serious possibilities. If the serious options have been excluded but the diagnosis is still not certain, it may be necessary to order diagnostic tests. This process forms part of Competency 1, 'Assess the patient'. An important decision at this point is whether to order diagnostic testing immediately or wait a couple of days (or even up to a week) to see how the symptoms and physical signs progress or perhaps settle. This 'watchful waiting' is common practice and a recognised diagnostic tool involving active monitoring of the condition in anticipation of a spontaneous resolution.

Differential diagnosis

Differential diagnosis is also part of Competency 1, 'Assess the patient'. The specific statement is 'makes, confirms or understands, the working or final diagnosis by systematically considering the various possibilities (differential diagnosis)'.

The processes described thus far cover differentiating; the next important step is to consider the actual diagnosis. In some cases, the cause of the patient's problem may be immediately obvious, due to the classic symptoms the patient is presenting. However, there may be a number of possibilities (differentials) and it is the clinician's job to distinguish between two or more by narrowing them down. This involves observing signs (such as raised blood pressure) and symptoms (such as headache) and putting them together to formulate more questions which will help narrow down the possibilities and come to a diagnosis.

The practitioner should ask the patient about any currently presenting symptoms, including any that started some time ago but that the patient feels may be related. Some symptoms (such as anxiety, pain and fatigue) are, by their nature, subjective. Constitutional symptoms are general symptoms that affect the entire body, such as unintentional weight loss, or shivers and aches experienced in flu-like illness. Signs, on the other hand, are objective and are observed by someone other than the patient – for example, a raised temperature or high blood pressure. However, these observed signs, linked to the patient's subjective symptoms, may still relate to more than one condition. In this case, a differential diagnosis is required, in which the practitioner first asks what is the most likely explanation; then, if it's not that, what else could it be?

The practitioner's reasoning ability enables them to make deductions based on the data gathered (history, presenting features, examination and investigation findings) to narrow down the different potential causes of the patient's presenting complaint. In addition, a degree of intuition and instinct often come into play in reaching a working diagnosis. Tacit knowledge cannot be taught and is a feature of expert diagnostic practice (Lymn *et al.* 2010). Diagnosis therefore means determining the nature of a disorder or problem by taking into account the patient's signs and symptoms, their medical history and (where necessary) any tests and physical examinations.

Diagnostic reasoning

Problem-solving and decision-making involve diagnostic reasoning based on intuition and knowledge. Sometimes it is impossible to reach an absolute diagnosis. In such cases, the practitioner's level of experience may increase the probability of a correct assumption.

Eventually, with experience and working in a narrow specialist area, the thought process needed for diagnosis will become largely subconscious. Prescribers will be aware of the clinical and geographic area in which they are practising. They will also know the age group of the patients being dealt with, and therefore the likelihood of a particular diagnosis based on signs and symptoms. In other words, they will be using the probability of a diagnosis to inform their decision. Further investigations and experience will improve that probability.

Nevertheless, all clinicians suffer from uncertainty. They have a limited time to carry out a consultation but, as long as they can rule out the serious possibilities quickly, they can wait until test results are obtained and arrange to see the patient again. If the patient's case needs to be discussed at a multidisciplinary meeting, the practitioner should be frank with the patient about this; it's safer for both the patient and the prescriber.

In summary, the competent practitioner acts on cues and identifies the most important signs and symptoms, and the most likely causes. The whole of Competency 1, 'Assess the patient', covers these aspects of the prescribing process (RPS 2016; see Appendix). The patient is the expert in describing the onset of the symptoms and what makes them worse or better. The pharmacist prescriber may have to undertake a physical examination to rule out possible conditions or disorders. The prescriber should also be able to use common diagnostic aids such as a sphygmomanometer and this is part of any prescribing course. Tests should be used as necessary, when unsure which of a number of possibilities is correct. The prescriber needs to be able to rule out serious conditions by looking for the absence of findings frequently seen in the condition. Using the subjective and objective information obtained, they should be able to see a pattern. In some cases, they may only be able to rule out a specific condition after an initial treatment and a review of the patient.

There are several excellent texts that go through each body system or clinical area, considering the various possibilities and ways of reducing uncertainty. For example, Dains *et al.* (2015) has a useful section which details differential diagnoses in a table format, thus providing a quick-reference summary of possible diagnoses for each patient problem. Texts like this, used in specific clinical areas, can improve confidence and lead to better diagnoses – or, at the very least, offer advice on what to do next in order to narrow down the possibilities and lead to a diagnosis.

Risk management

Shimizu *et al.* (2012) found that the use of a differential diagnosis checklist enhanced diagnostic performance in complex cases, with the intuitive process remaining superior in less difficult cases. Based on what has been said before, the general checklist for diagnosis would be:

- Obtain a complete medical history
- Carry out a purposeful and focused physical examination
- Generate initial hypotheses and differentiate these with additional questions, physical examination and diagnostic tests
- Pause to reflect – take diagnostic time out
  - Was I comprehensive?
  - Did I consider the flaws of heuristic thinking?
  - Was my judgement affected by any other bias?
  - Do I need to make the diagnosis now or can it wait?
  - What is the worst-case scenario?
- Embark on a plan but acknowledge uncertainty and ensure there is a pathway for follow-up investigations.

Discussing the likely diagnosis

Following any physical examination findings or further tests, conclusions need to be discussed with the patient. All patients are different; the level and amount of information they want will also differ. There is a duty to explain clearly and truthfully what the diagnosis is believed to be and also what the treatment options are. It is the prescriber's job to ascertain how much and at what level the information to be discussed should be. Using patient information leaflets or providing evidence-based patient websites for the patient to visit later can enhance their comprehension of the condition which in turn may enable a greater understanding and involvement with choosing between treatment options.

Working with the patient to plan management

At this point, the recommended options for management should be discussed. These options may be narrow or broad, depending on the diagnosis and whether there is a need for immediate pharmacological intervention. This stage relates to Competency 2 ('Consider the options') and 3 ('Reach a shared decision'). For example, a patient with a lower respiratory chest infection should commence immediate antibiotic treatment with careful observation, whereas a patient with Type 2 diabetes will require an approach tailored to their signs and symptoms.

Watchful waiting is the best policy in some circumstances prior to ordering tests, and the same principle can also be applied at this juncture. For instance, the patient may appear to have a self-limiting condition, such as heartburn or indigestion, and conservative measures and self-help strategies (including visiting the pharmacy) might be suggested. Similarly, a safety-netting approach might involve issuing a prescription which is only to be used if symptoms do not improve after a specific time period (Neighbour 2005). If this approach is suggested and the patient agrees, it is important to be very clear regarding the expected outcome and the need to return if the condition deteriorates or doesn't improve. The pharmacist prescriber must always know their own limitations. If any deterioration or change in the patient's condition lies outside the prescriber's scope of competence, the patient should be given advice on whom to see at a future appointment.

Establishing the clinical purpose of prescribing

There are 14 elements to Competency 4 ('Prescribe), all of which need careful consideration. If 'watchful waiting' is not an option, and prescribing a drug treatment is the most appropriate course of action, the patient should be told about the expected outcome of the prescription. Obviously it would be preferable if all interventions were curative but many will offer only symptomatic relief. Indeed, symptomatic relief may be all that *can* be offered – for example, in age-related problems such as joint aches.

In some instances, prescribing will be tactical – when the recognised causes and treatments of a symptom have been exhausted and a possibility is being tested. Acid reflux may cause a persistent pithy cough, rather than the usual dyspeptic symptoms of indigestion or heartburn, and a trial of an H2-receptor antagonist or proton pump inhibitor will test this possibility. Tactical prescribing can also be employed while waiting for results from tests – for instance, treating a rash with an antifungal cream while awaiting mycology results from skin scrapings.

In the case of antibiotic interventions (which are mainly curative, though they can be used as prophylaxis before some types of surgery), treatment may sometimes be empirical, though certain empirical treatment assumptions have proven to be robust. For instance, in the case of women with urgency, frequency and dysuria, these symptoms give a 95% post-symptom probability for uncomplicated cystitis (Baerheim 2012). On many occasions, the therapeutic intervention will be prophylactic or preventative, as in migraine treatments, gout, or giving antimalarial prophylaxis.

Finally, the medication choice may modify the disease, as with disease-modifying anti-rheumatic drugs (DMARDs). Being clear about the clinical purpose of prescribing is important, not only in terms of growing as a prescriber but also in enhancing the prescriber's ability to communicate the therapeutic aims of treatment to patients. A fully informed patient is more likely to agree to commence and adhere to suggested treatment, and therefore more likely to improve in response to that treatment.

Making joint decisions

Competency 3 ('Reach a shared decision') has been discussed above. Armed with a clear therapeutic purpose for prescribing, based on the patient's profile and comorbidities, current medications and drug allergies, it will be possible to choose and recommend the most suitable drug(s). National guidelines, such as NICE and SIGN, should be the theoretical backbone of practice, complemented by resources that provide information on the practical application of particular types of medication.

It is best to have a relatively small armamentarium. Reliable, regularly updated sources of information are needed to ensure that prescribers are aware of any changes in the clinical area. If working in hospital, practitioners will be expected to prescribe within the formulary agreed by the Medicines Committee/Drug and Therapeutics Committees. All prescribers have a professional duty to be up to date in their particular specialist area. To this end, they should identify authoritative, evidence-based websites to refer to.

For example, one major website is medicines.org.uk (Datapharm 2019). This has the patient information leaflet (PIL) as well as the Summary of Product Characteristics (SmPC). The PIL can be printed out to go through with the patient, and this may generate questions which can be answered immediately, during the consultation. Competency 5 is 'Provide information' and statement 5.3 is 'guides patients/carers on how to identify reliable sources of information about their medicines and treatments'. Once the information has been seen, the patient may therefore want to find out more. In this case, the prescriber may wish to suggest appropriate websites, such as patient.info (Patient Platform 2019). This site is particularly useful as it has sections for health professionals as well as patient information sections. In general practice and primary care, there are a number of sites such as GP Notebook (Oxbridge Solutions Ltd 2019), which is an excellent succinct resource.

If this is the first time the patient has had this medication, there may be quite a lot to explain. Obviously, the prescription is only one part of a package of care. For example, if the medication is for a joint pain, losing weight may be beneficial or, in some cases, specific exercises could help. For the latter, a referral to a physiotherapist may be considered. If necessary, diagrams may help understanding and recall (NICE 2009). It is useful to talk to patients about the benefits, likely outcomes and potential side effects of drugs, and also – most importantly – to establish whether or not the patient agrees to the treatment. If this is latter point is not ascertained, the whole consultation could end up being a waste of time. This is a marker of patient-centeredness; is the patient satisfied and happy with the plan? If the strategies recommended in this chapter are employed, the power will probably have been balanced equally between the prescriber and the patient. According to Jagosh *et al.* (2011), trust evolves as a consequence of a good practitioner–patient relationship, and this good relationship can lead to patients being more satisfied with decisions and therefore being more likely to adhere to recommended treatment.

In some cases, the patient's agenda may not have been met. This is often (but not always) associated with antibiotics and the public health duty in antibiotic stewardship. These and other public health duties are discussed later in Chapter 4.

Closing the consultation and record-keeping

Competency 6 ('Monitor and review') concludes the consultation. Having agreed the forward treatment plan, the prescriber should now cover any health promotion and disease prevention recommendations (if they haven't already been included in earlier discussions about treatment).

These discussions highlight the fact that the patient has responsibility for their own health and enables the practitioner to offer support for other aspects of the patient's condition.

It's a good idea to suggest timescales for review, to ensure that outcomes are as expected; these will vary, depending on the condition and the recommended treatment. If the condition improves as anticipated, the patient may be advised that there is no need for review. However, if treatment is not effective within a given timeframe or the condition deteriorates, it's important to have a clear plan of action for review, either with the original prescriber or with other members of staff or other out-of-hour services.

It should be emphasised that initial treatment plans are based on the current state of the patient's condition, which may change over time and an amended or completely different approach may therefore be required. Common side effects will have been discussed earlier but they need to be reiterated at this point to help the patient remember what they might be and what to do if they develop. This final 'safety netting' stage is a good way of closing the consultation.

Competency 4 ('Prescribe') includes 4.12: 'makes accurate legible and contemporaneous records and clinical notes of prescribing decisions' (RPS 2016; see Appendix). It is essential to make contemporaneous notes as soon as possible after the conclusion of the consultation. The maxim 'if it isn't written down, it didn't happen' (Editorial 2013) should be borne in mind by all prescribers. Keeping appropriately detailed records is essential, not only for the original prescriber but also for the next prescriber or practitioner, as the patient may see other practitioners, who will need to be able to refer to an up-to-date patient record. Write sufficiently detailed notes so as to remember why particular decisions were made, including the rationale for these decisions. This is particularly important if a treatment plan was agreed which better meets the patient's ICEs but is outside local or national recommendations.

Influences on the pharmacist prescriber

It is important to acknowledge that prescribing does not take place in a vacuum. Many influences can affect pharmacist prescribers. For instance, pharmaceutical companies may try to encourage the prescriber to move to their product or there may be financial restraints that encourage the prescriber to use cheaper products. These influences can be minimised by the use of formularies, local trust guidelines and primary care organisations. Medicines are one of the most common healthcare interventions, and prescribers may not always be aware of the many influences on their prescribing habits and decisions.

Personal influences

There may be personal influences, based on the prescriber's beliefs and prejudices – for example, when deciding whether or not to offer contraception or IVF. The prescriber's views on drug abuse could influence decisions about prescribing certain drugs. Personal views and beliefs about prescribing for conditions linked to lifestyle (such as obesity) may also influence prescribing decisions.

The six short statements making up Competency 3, 'Reach a shared decision' (RPS 2016; see Appendix), include the principle that prescribing decisions should be based on the needs of patients and not on the prescriber's personal considerations. The biggest personal influence is likely to be a lack of confidence, which can be overcome by continuing professional development

(CPD) and experience. It is a key competency for a prescriber to understand their own limitations and know when more information, support or guidance is needed, or even when to refer to another prescriber. Competency 7 ('Prescribe safely') and Competency 8 ('Prescribe professionally') look at prescribing governance, including recognising limits and skills (RPS 2016; see Appendix).

External influences on prescribing

Patients can sometimes make demands of prescribers, suggesting what they need based on their own experience. Prescribers shouldn't dismiss patients' comments, as they need all the information they can get (for more on this, see Chapter 2 on communication). However, we shouldn't always assume that a patient wants a prescription. In a study of 544 consultations, 25% of patients who wanted a prescription did not get one, 30% of those who did not want a prescription did receive one and 22% of prescriptions were given for reasons other than purely a clinical indication. Doctors were more likely to prescribe if they felt pressurised and if they perceived that the patient expected a prescription (Britten & Ukoumunne 1997).

Media influence

Patients may seek advice after they have gathered information on possible treatments from newspaper reports or online sources. It is difficult to keep up with all emerging media reports on medications but prescribers need to be aware that this may happen. Medicine information in various formats is available and should be used. Always consider the risks and benefits of any new treatment, or of established treatments being used in unfamiliar ways. The patient may be concerned that they have a condition that is being discussed in the media, or the treatment they have tried before may not have been successful and they require further help. Competency 3 ('Reach a shared decision') includes the requirement to work with the patient/carer to make informed choices that respect patient preferences, including their right to refuse or limit treatment (see Chapter 2 for a discussion of types of consultation).

Industrial influences

There are many ways in which the pharmaceutical industry tries to influence prescribers. The obvious ones are through drug company representatives, journal advertisements and mailings. A House of Commons Select Committee report (2005) suggests:

> The blame for inadequate or misinformed prescribing decisions does not only lie with the pharmaceutical industry, but with doctors and other prescribers who do not keep abreast of medicines information and are sometimes too willing to accept hospitality from the industry and act uncritically on the information supplied by the drug companies.

The drug company representative

There are approximately 8,000 drug company representatives operating in the UK. They visit GPs and hospitals, though the regulation in hospital is often more rigorous. The representative is a two-way influence. They bring information about new drugs or new applications for old drugs; they maintain the sales and position of established drugs; and they offer an information service, taking back queries to the company who employs them. New drugs are often massively promoted when they first come out. The representative will try to ensure that hospital consultants are familiar with the new treatment because of the potential influence of consultants on general practice prescribing. Representatives may also contact patient groups and primary care organisations; prescribing committees may well have these informed patients on their boards.

Professional influences

There are also, of course, professional influences, including budgetary constraints. Those in charge of formularies, particularly in hospitals, will try to ensure that the most cost-effective medicines are used and prescribed. Any pharmacist prescriber in the community needs to think very carefully before prescribing any new drug. Guidance from pharmaceutical advisers in clinical commissioning groups (CCGs), Health Boards and Trusts in the United Kingdom should be taken very seriously. Prescribers in general practice may find that the hospital consultants may wish to try to influence them to prescribe drugs that are not on the hospital formulary.

Prescribing analyses

In the community, prescriptions are centralised for payments so all prescriptions dispensed are added to a database; this makes it possible to analyse prescribing and spot trends in the data. Prescribing analyses are essential tools for advisers, and pharmacist prescribers' prescribing will form part of the database, alongside that of doctors, dentists, nurses and any others where the prescriptions are dispensed by community pharmacies or dispensing doctors and a small number of specialist appliance suppliers and stoma providers.

Advisers can manipulate the data to show the results for one practice versus another, or individual practices versus an average for the area, or even individual practices versus an agreed level of use. Different primary care areas can be compared with national averages, or with other primary care organisations with similar demographics. Levels of generic prescribing can be identified and the analyses can be used to guide and support prescribers and to inform a prescribing discussion meeting. A detailed analysis of prescribing analyses throughout the United Kingdom is beyond the scope of this short book but those undertaking medicines management or optimisation will be able to help. Such analyses can be an important influence on prescribers as they can help them to reflect on their prescribing decisions.

How can we ensure that the influences on prescribing are appropriate and evidence-based? Probably the most important way to ensure that influences are kept to a minimum is for prescribers to become knowledgeable about the drugs that are commonly prescribed. This is one reason why it has been suggested that new pharmacist prescribers should specialise in a particular area and then they can get to know the range of medicines well. Obviously, it is essential to ensure that all claims made for any medicines are checked; prescribers should generally be sceptical.

Continuing education and continuing professional development are also essential. Conferences, professional meetings and medicines information committees can all be useful, though time-consuming. There may be a local network of pharmacist prescribers. If so, such a network can offer support, particularly for those who are new to prescribing. The internet gives access to a massive medical information database (as mentioned earlier). Prescribers should also ensure that at least some of their CPD is related to prescribing and keeping up to date. Reading, writing papers and giving lectures can all form part of this.

If working in an Acute Trust, there are likely to be formularies and Trust guidance. Other decision support systems such as clinical knowledge summaries (CKS), available through NICE, are useful for practical guidance on treatments. Medicines information units in the local Trust can usually answer queries about medicines; and, if not, they have access to specialist units around the country. Prescribers should get to know experts, pharmacists, nurses or doctors and make contact with them. National bodies that specialise in areas such as Diabetes UK or the Alzheimer's Society have information that can be helpful in their areas and can discuss issues of concern with regard to prescribing in those areas. Recognise that prescribers are responsible for what they prescribe but also that they can be influenced – and that influence should be based on the national guidance wherever possible.

Summary

It has been argued that the patient consultation, including observing signs and symptoms, is the most important aspect of prescribing. In this chapter, different models of consultation have been considered, and the attitudes and behaviours needed to pursue a patient-centred approach have been discussed. Influences on prescribers have been briefly explored and ways of minimising these suggested. All prescribers are susceptible to being influenced.

Having read this chapter, it may be concluded that a patient-centred consultation could take a very long time. However, with experience, it will become second nature and the prescriber will be able to skilfully listen, question, analyse and negotiate a management plan in the expected timescale. Further theories to inform patient-centred practice will be discussed in Chapter 4, which focuses on adherence with the central aim of placing the patient's best interest at the centre of decision-making.

References

Baerheim, A. (2012). Empirical treatment of uncomplicated cystitis. *Scandinavian Journal of Primary Health Care*. **30**, 1–2.

Barker, L.R., Burton, J. R. & Zieve, P.D. (2007) *Principles of Ambulatory Medicine*. 7th edn. Philadelphia USA: Lippincott, Williams and Wilkin.

Birks, Y. & Watt, I. (2007). Emotional intelligence and patient-centred care. *Journal of the Royal Society of Medicine*. **100**, 369–74.

Britten, N. & Ukoumunne, O. (1997). The influence of patient's hopes of receiving a prescription on doctors' perceptions and the decision to prescribe: a questionnaire study. *British Medical Journal* **315**,1506–10

Bub, B. (2004). The patient's lament: hidden key to effective communication: how to recognise and transform. *Medical Humanities*. **30**, 63–69.

Chew, K.S., Jeroen, J.G. *et al.* (2016). A portable mnemonic to facilitate checking for cognitive errors. *BMC Research Notes*. **9**(1).

Dains, J.E., Baumann, L.C. & Scheibel, P. (2015). *Advanced Health Assessment and Clinical Diagnosis in Primary Care*. 5th edn. St. Louis, Missouri, USA: Elsevier.

Datapharm (2019). *Electronic Medicine Compendium*. https://www.medicines.org.uk/emc (last accessed 16.5.2019).

Deveugele, M.A., Derese, D. *et al.* (2004). Consultation in general practice: a standard operating procedure? *Patient Education and Counselling*. **54**(2), 227–33.

Dowie, J. & Elstein, A. (1988) *Professional Judgement. A reader in clinical decision-making*. Cambridge: Cambridge University Press.

Editorial (2013). Would your records stand up to scrutiny? *Nursing Times*.

Fraser. R. (ed) (1999). *Clinical method: A general practice approach*. 3rd edn. Oxford: Butterworth Heinemann.

Fulop, M. (1985). Teaching differential diagnosis to beginning clinical students. *The American Journal of Medicine.* **79**(6), 745–49.

General Pharmaceutical Council (GPhC) (2016). *Prescribers Survey Report*. https://www.pharmacyregulation.org/sites/default/files/gphc_prescribers_survey_report.pdf (last accessed 14.5.2019).

General Pharmaceutical Council (GPhC) (2017). *Standards for pharmacy professionals* https://www.pharmacyregulation.org/spp (last accessed 17.5.2019).

Gill, C. & Murphy, M. (2014). 'Communication and patient collaboration' In: B. Strickland-Hodge & H. Bradbury (eds) *Practical prescribing for medical students*. London: SAGE Publications.

Gillard, S., Benson, J. & Silverman, J. 2009. Teaching and assessment of explanation and planning in medical schools in the United Kingdom: cross sectional questionnaire survey. *Medical Teacher.* **31**(4), 328–31.

Gray, D. & Toghill, P. (eds) (2000). *Introduction to the Symptoms and Signs of Clinical Medicine: A Hands-on Guide to Developing Core Skills*. London: Hodder Arnold.

Hampton, J.R., Harrison, M.J., *et al.* (1975). Relative contributions of history-taking, physical examination, and laboratory investigation to diagnosis and management of medical outpatients. *British Medical Journal.* **2**(5969), 486–89.

House of Commons (2005). *Select committee report on the pharmaceutical industry*. London: Stationery Office. https://publications.parliament.uk/pa/cm200405/cmselect/cmhealth/42/42.pdf (last accessed 17.5.2019).

Jagosh, J., Donald Boudreau, J., *et al.* (2011). The importance of physician listening from the patients' perspective: enhancing diagnosis, healing, and the doctor-patient relationship. *Patient Education and Counselling.* **85**(3), 369–74.

Kurtz, S., Silverman, J., *et al.* (2003). Marrying content and process in clinical method teaching; Enhancing the Calgary-Cambridge Guides. *Academic Medicine.* 78, 8. http://www.gp-training.net/training/communication_skills/calgary/framwork/framework.htm http://www.gp-training.net/ (last accessed 17.5.2019).

Lado, E., Vacariza, M. *et al.* (2008). Influence extended on drug prescribing by patients' attitudes and expectations and by doctors' perception of such expectations: a cohort and nested case-control study. *Journal of Evaluation in Clinical Practice.* **14**(3), 453–59.

Lymn, J., Bowskill, D., Bath-Hextall & Knagggs, R. (2010). *The New Prescriber: an integrated approach to medical and non-medical prescribing*. 1st edn. Chichester: Wiley, Blackwell.

Matthys, J., Elwyn, G. *et al.* (2009). Patients' ideas, concerns, and expectations (ICE) in general practice: impact on prescribing. *British Journal of General Practice.* **59**(558), 29–36.

McEwen, A. & Harris, G. (2010). 'Chapter 1 Communication: fundamental skills' In: *Communication Skills for Adult Nurses*. New York USA: McGraw-Hill Education

Mechanic, D. (ed.) (1982). *Symptoms, illness behavior, and help-seeking*. New Brunswick, New Jersey: Rutgers University Press.

Medicines and Healthcare products Regulatory Agency (MHRA) (2019). *Medicines Information: SPCs & PILs*. http://www.mhra.gov.uk/spc-pil/index.htm (last accessed 15.5.2019).

Moulton, L. (2007). *The Naked Consultation: A Practical Guide to Primary Care Consultation Skills*. London: Radcliffe Publishing Ltd.

Mustafa, M., Wood, F. *et al.* (2014). Managing expectations of antibiotics for upper respiratory tract infections: A qualitative study. *Annals of Family Medicine.* **12**(1), 29–36.

National Institute for Health and Care Excellence (NICE) (2009). Medicines Adherence: involving patients in decisions about prescribed medicines and supporting adherence. *NICE Clinical Guideline* **76**. London: NICE.

Neighbour, R. (2005). *The inner consultation: How to develop an effective and intuitive consulting style*. 2nd edn. Oxford: Radcliffe.

Nickless, G. & Noble, H. (2009) How to take an accurate medication history when a patient is admitted. *Clinical Pharmacist*. Pharmaceutical Journal, Royal Pharmaceutical Society.

Oxbridge Solutions Ltd (2019). *GP Notebook*. http://www.gpnotebook.co.uk/homepage.cfm (last accessed 16.5.2019).

Patient Platform Ltd (2019). https://patient.info (last accessed 16.5.2019).

Royal Pharmaceutical Society (RPS) (2016). *A Competency Framework for All Prescribers*. London: RPS. https://www.rpharms.com/Portals/0/RPS%20document%20library/Open%20access/Professional%20standards/Prescribing%20competency%20framework/prescribing-competency-framework.pdf (last accessed 14.5.2019).

Schwartz, A. & Bergus, G. (2008). *Medical decision making: a physician's guide.* Cambridge: Cambridge University Press.

Shimizu, T., Matsumoto, K. & Tokuda, Y. (2012). Effects of the use of differential diagnosis checklist and general de-biasing checklist on diagnostic performance in comparison to intuitive diagnosis. *Medical Teacher.* **35**(6).

Silverman, D. (2014). *Interpreting Qualitative Data Methods for Analysing Talk.* 3rd edn. London: Sage Publications.

3

Patient clinical assessment

Catherine Gill

Chapter overview

This chapter presents a taster of physical examination skills, clinical assessment and general common physical signs of ill health. It should be used in conjunction with the examination skills taught on any relevant in-house or external course and while working within the usual team. If they are in a prescribing role, pharmacists are expected to examine patients regularly; and it is recommended that they should at least undertake a further module in clinical reasoning and physical assessment in order to fulfil such a specialist role. This chapter briefly considers the issue of pharmacists' clinical assessment of patients.

It also covers the skills needed to assess the patient's status in the following areas: the respiratory domain (including pulse oximetry and capillary refill), temperature, pulse and blood pressure and general common physical signs of ill health. Finally, the chapter discusses the assessment skills required to monitor and identify the deteriorating patient using the National Early Warning Score Tool (NEWS) 2 Table 4 (RCP 2017).

Introduction

Within any prescribing programme, there will be a taught component covering physical examination but this will only be an introduction and the practitioner will also need to be assessed in the workplace as competent if the role requires this skill set. This will cover a minimum standard and pharmacist prescribers may need to undertake additional patient assessments and diagnostic reasoning modules/programme(s) to ensure that they are competent to undertake the role of prescriber. As described earlier, the *Prescribers Survey Report* suggested that respondents felt they lacked clinical assessment skills after qualifying and they did not always feel confident in diagnosing. It was also highlighted that pharmacist responders did not generally receive opportunities to develop physical assessment skills as part of their training (GPhC 2016). It is hoped that this situation will improve as undergraduate pharmacy courses in the UK increase their clinical component and involve patients more. The fact that the Independent Prescribing (IP) courses all now have an assessed element of clinical examination should also be helpful.

In the *Competency Framework for All Prescribers* (RPS 2016; see Appendix), it is suggested that a clinical assessment needs to be undertaken by the independent prescriber. However, the definition of independent prescribing includes 'diagnosed or undiagnosed conditions'. Independent prescribing is:

- Prescribing by an appropriate practitioner (e.g. a doctor, dentist, nurse, pharmacist, etc.) who is responsible and accountable for the assessment of patients with undiagnosed or diagnosed conditions and for decisions about the clinical management required, including prescribing.

There are specific points within the framework. For instance, Competency 1 ('Assess the patient') includes statement 1.2: 'undertakes an appropriate clinical assessment'. The word 'appropriate' is important here and suggests that pharmacists in a very narrow specialist area of practice should be able to perform the appropriate clinical assessment themselves, while those in general practice may need to start work following a diagnosis and clinical assessment by other practitioners.

Also, in Competency 1, statement 1.8 includes the phrase: 'refers to or seeks guidance from another member of the team, a specialist or a prescribing information source when necessary'. In Competency 7, 'Prescribe safely', statements such as 7.1 ('prescribes within own scope of practice and recognises the limits of own knowledge and skill') are stressed, so that the pharmacist realises that they should refer to another member of the team if they do not feel competent to undertake the clinical assessment themselves.

Competency 10 ('Prescribe as part of a team') reminds the pharmacist that they should work closely with colleagues to maintain their own identity as pharmacists, while ensuring that they utilise their colleagues' experience and knowledge which may be in the clinical assessment of patients. This is highlighted in the framework with statements such as 10.1 ('acts as part of a multidisciplinary team to ensure that continuity of care across care settings is developed and not compromised'), 10.2 ('establishes relationships with other professionals based on understanding, trust, respect for each other's roles in relation to prescribing') and 10.3 ('negotiates the appropriate level of support and supervision for role as a prescriber'). All this guidance helps the independent pharmacist prescriber to fulfil the prescribing role while maintaining patient safety and ensuring the best outcomes for patients.

The original learning outcomes, approved by the General Pharmaceutical Council (undated) and the Nursing and Midwifery Council, state:

> Describe the pathophysiology of the condition being treated and recognise the signs and symptoms of illness, take an accurate history and carry out a relevant clinical assessment where necessary.

> Use common diagnostic aids e.g. stethoscope, sphygmomanometer.

> Use diagnostic aids relevant to the condition(s) for which the pharmacist intends to prescribe, including monitoring response to therapy.

The learning outcomes indicate that the qualified pharmacist prescriber should be able to apply clinical assessment skills to:

- Inform a working diagnosis
- Formulate a treatment plan
- Prescribe one or more medicines if appropriate

- Carry out a checking process to ensure patient safety
- Monitor response to therapy, review the working/differential diagnosis and modify treatment or refer/consult/seek guidance as appropriate.

Finally, as with the framework mentioned above, the learning outcomes state:

- Demonstrate a shared approach to decision making by assessing patients' needs for medicines, taking account of their wishes and values and those of their carers when making prescribing decisions.

The curriculum for the undergraduate MPharm degree, as outlined in the 2011 document, Future pharmacists: Standards for the initial education and training of pharmacists' (GPhC 2011), states that the newly qualified graduate should be able to identify and employ the appropriate diagnostic or physiological testing techniques to inform clinical decision-making, which is already part of prescribing courses. In the document, as part of the indicative syllabus, A1.2 'How people work', it also states the following series of objectives:

- Diagnosis
- Differential diagnosis
- Symptom recognition
- Diagnostic tests.

As the basics of clinical assessment are included in the MPharm, this process will have been introduced and can be developed during the pre-registration year and the following years as required.

As stated in earlier chapters, the GPhC commissioned a *Prescribers Survey Report* (GPhC 2016) and subsequent reports to identify areas of strength and potential concern for new prescribers. By becoming prescribers, pharmacists have an opportunity to expand their role and take on all aspects of the patient journey, from diagnosis to prescribing, advice and follow-up.

The *Prescribers Survey Report* made a number of statements that are relevant to this chapter. For example (GPhC 2016, p. 5, para 1.10):

> Despite their expertise in medicines, we heard that respondents could feel they lacked clinical assessment skills after qualifying and that they did not always feel confident in diagnosing. It was highlighted that pharmacists do not generally receive opportunities to develop physical assessment skills as part of their training. However this lack of confidence in assessment could be addressed through working alongside others within the multi-disciplinary team, such as nurses, who were felt to have more clinical experience through training.

There were a few comments about the lack of clinical assessment skills, especially early on in prescribers' careers, and how this could be problematic for pharmacist prescribers. However, the definition of independent prescribing includes undiagnosed patients as well as those already diagnosed who have undergone a clinical assessment. Newly qualified pharmacist prescribers should work within their own limitations and as part of a team. While pharmacists were referred to as experts in medicines, nurses and doctors were felt to have more training and experience in diagnosis. Their diagnostic skill has largely come from experience with patients, and this clinical experience is what the pharmacist needs most (GPhC 2016, p. 7, para 2.12):

One of the key differences of the pharmacist independent prescriber role, over the pharmacist supplementary prescriber role, is that the former can make a diagnosis for the patient concerned and can prescribe independently to them, without the need to consult other independent prescribers; whereas the latter can only prescribe within the framework of a patient-specific clinical management plan, agreed by a doctor or dentist.

In which areas should the independent pharmacist feel competent? Firstly, they should be able to recognise red flags (those signs, symptoms or conditions that make it essential to seek advice, a second opinion or support). These red flags are discussed a little later in this chapter. Secondly, they should have an understanding of differential diagnosis and how to narrow down from a broad overview to a specific area of concern.

The 2016 survey went on to discuss clinical knowledge and skills. There was substantial feedback on this area, particularly on clinical assessment skill (GPhC 2016, p. 15, para 4.10):

> An issue on which we received feedback was in relation to clinical assessment skills. A number of respondents reported that they lacked such skills and did not feel confident in making initial diagnoses. This feedback should be understood in the context of changes to pharmacist training more broadly – the MPharm does have more emphasis on clinical skills so this is likely to be less of an issue for newly graduating pharmacists.

However, it will depend on the way the clinical assessment is taught and assessed and the time devoted to it. As mentioned above, pharmacists are charged with ensuring they practise within their scope of professional and clinical competence. As a 'trainee' prescriber, there are physical assessment competencies and curricula which must be assessed (GPhC 2012). The basic physical examination skills taught and assessed will depend on the particular university attended. However, in all universities, competency is assessed using the *Competency Framework for all Prescribers* (RPS 2016; see Appendix). Physical examination skills will initially be acquired in a simulated environment, progressing to a clinical setting.

Overall evaluation and the measurement of vital signs are the most vital aspects of assessing and monitoring patients' physiological status. Following university and practising in the simulated environment, pharmacists need to practise in the clinical setting until they have learnt and mastered each skill. In order to do this, they need to be aware of each vital sign parameter – that is, the reference ranges which are considered normal. Vital signs outside these reference ranges may be classed as abnormal but, when found in isolation, may not be clinically significant. Decisions about a patient's treatment are often based on overall trends and the whole clinical picture. As discussed in Chapter 2, much of clinical conjecture is based on the history with which the patient presents. A thorough and detailed history will help to structure and guide the clinical examination.

Pre-examination procedure

Before undertaking a clinical examination, the patient's permission and consent must be gained, and a brief explanation of the physical examination procedure should be given. Measures must be taken to ensure privacy and confidentiality and a chaperone should be offered. Whether or not the patient accepts the offer of a chaperone should be documented in the patient's notes (GPhC

2012). Hands must be washed and sterilised. Although this should be the norm, unfortunately it is not always the case and, according to the National Institute for Health and Care Excellence (NICE 2017), many healthcare-related infections are due to poor hand hygiene on the part of healthcare professionals. Ensure the patient is comfortable before the assessment begins.

Red flags and the initial consultation

General inspection

On first contact with the patient, a quick general inspection should be made, noting whether they look unwell, distressed or in pain. Are they cachectic (i.e. malnourished and emaciated with sunken cheeks and general physical wasting)? Are they breathless? Can they speak comfortably or are they struggling to complete a sentence without breaking to take a breath every second or third word? Do they appear confused, agitated or drowsy? Do they have any evidence of sudden loss of function or facial palsy (weakness)? Is there oedema of the face, sacral area or lower limbs indicating a cardiovascular or hepatic or general allergic response? Are they dressed appropriately for the weather and environment? Do they have any obvious medical needs (such as any sign of bleeding)? Once it has been determined that urgent medical assistance is not required, a more structured assessment can be undertaken as follows.

General assessment

Simply watching the patient breathe can yield a wealth of information. Observe the general ease of breathing, noting if the breaths are regular and within normal limits (see Table 3.2 for normal reference ranges). Alternatively, is the breathing laboured, involving the use of accessory muscles of breathing (commonly scalenes, sternomastoids, abdominals, intercostals)?

Note how the patient is sitting (the position assumed), as this is an important indicator of both acute and chronic respiratory dysfunction. For example, respiratory-challenged patients will naturally sit forward, supporting themselves with their hands braced on their knees – the tripod position. This is an unconscious physiological adaptation to disarranged blood gases. Sitting forward helps the diaphragm to move lower; the lungs then have an increased area to expand into and this can facilitate gas exchange. Pursed lipped breathing (PLB) is another example of unconscious physiological adaptation, in which the patient purses the lips on expiration. (Note that not all patients have this unconscious adaptation and may have to be taught the technique in pulmonary rehabilitation.) PLB is thought to prevent tightness in the airway by providing resistance to expiration and has been shown to increase the use of the diaphragm and decrease accessory muscle recruitment.

Skin tone

Does the patient appear unusually pale, which could indicate anaemia or activation of the sympathetic arm of the autonomic nervous system? Does their skin have a bluish tint, which could suggest central cyanosis? Or does their skin have a yellow discoloration, which may be suggestive of a liver disorder? Inspection of the sclera and conjunctiva of the eye will help diagnose anaemia and jaundice. Unexplained pallor and central cyanosis are red flags and assistance should be summoned immediately. Conditions such as hypothyroid disorders, and liver or renal disease can lead to thin skin, while acromegaly produces overly thick skin. Check for any obvious rash and remember that the presence of a non-blanching rash requires urgent medical assessment.

Face

The assessment begins with a general appraisal, observing the patient's overall facial symmetry at rest. Are there any involuntary movements, facial tics or fasciculation? These might simply be a manifestation of stress and anxiety or they could have a neurological cause. As the patient blinks, is there any delay on one side? If so, are there any other differences on the same side, such as a flatter nasolabial fold or the mouth drooping at the corner, more noticeable during smiling and less so when speaking? Facial palsy can be caused by several system disorders, including neurological, cerebrovascular, dystrophy or neuropathy. Is there normal hair distribution? Has the patient any hair loss (male pattern balding is normal in men) or general loss of bodily hair or an increase (such as excessive facial hair in a female) which may be indicative of an endocrine problem? Does the patient have a round moon face (so-called Cushingoid) as a result of long-term use of steroids or Cushing disease?

Eyes

Examine the external structures of the eyes for symmetry; both eyelids should cover roughly the same area of the eyeball. Any drooping of the lids (ptosis) may be age-related, as the levator muscle weakens and stretches over time, or it could be a result of damage to the nerves controlling these structures (cranial nerves 3 and 7). Other causes can be as simple as a local swelling, such as a stye, or more serious causes such as a tumour around or behind the eye, Horner's syndrome, myasthenia gravis or stroke.

Are there any fatty yellow deposits or lumps in the delicate skin around the eyes and eyelids, known as xanthelasma? This may be an idiopathic occurrence or it could be a sign of raised cholesterol and triglycerides. Observe the pupil and iris; normally both these structures are round and symmetrical. Note the white of the eye (the sclera) which surrounds the iris and pupil; a yellowish tinge or clear yellow staining is caused by a number of liver or blood disorders which lead to an excessive build-up of bilirubin (hyperbilirubinaemia). The reason for this could be gallstones, hepatitis, alcoholic liver disease, pancreatitis or sickle cell disease.

Is the conjunctiva transparent and clear or is the capillary network noticeable or 'bloodshot' (the medical term is 'injected')? Dilated blood vessels or injection can be caused by infection, allergy, a foreign body and irritation; all will result in conjunctivitis. A dense bright red area under the conjunctiva, a subconjunctival haemorrhage, can look very alarming but is usually not serious and often caused by coughing, sneezing or following straining. The patient's history should be checked: when did it occur and is there any other bleeding (such as nose bleeds) which might point towards a bleeding disorder? Blood pressure should be measured, as hypertension is a (rare) cause and anticoagulant medication use needs to be excluded as a possible cause. The conjunctiva also lines the inside of the eyelids, and the tissues of the inner lids are usually a light red colour (in anaemia they are pale). Permission to examine the patient's inner eyelid must be sought; then the little finger of the dominant hand should be used to gently expose the lower inner lid conjunctiva.

Mouth

Next, the patient's lips should be checked. What colour are the lips? Is there a blue tinge indicating peripheral cyanosis? Are the corners dry and or split? This is termed angular stomatitis. Iron and vitamin B12 deficiency can cause angular stomatitis, and a persistent stomatitis in the absence of anaemia can be a fungal infection. Are there any lesions indicative of herpes simplex or impetigo? The history will be of vesicles or blisters on or around the lips which have ulcerated then crusted. Are the lips dry or moist (dry lips can point to dehydration)? Or is there any swelling or oedema of the lips as a response to local or systemic allergy? Angio-oedema includes a swollen tongue so the patient should be asked to put out their tongue and if the tongue is also oedematous urgent medical assistance should be sought.

Other observations of the tongue include: is it dry or moist, cyanosed or discoloured? The presence of a blue tongue (central cyanosis) is a major red flag requiring urgent medical assistance. A dry furred hairy tongue can indicate reduced oral fluid intake and potential dehydration. A wrinkled fissured red-brown coloured tongue (referred to as a beef steak tongue) is suggestive of iron deficiency anaemia. The tongue epidermis is rough textured, with papillae that are dense at the tip and body of the tongue but larger with smooth areas at the root of the tongue.

Is there any loss of the normal papillary distribution of the tongue? A bright red smooth sore tongue can be associated with vitamin B12 deficiency and pernicious anaemia. White plaque-like lesions on the tongue or oral mucosa are likely to indicate oral candida and *can* be rubbed off (if this is seen on the oral mucosa, a gauze can be used to try to rub it off). Leucoplakia will *not* rub off and has pre-malignant potential – the patient should be immediately directed to the dentist to have a biopsy.

While inspecting the tongue, note the patient's breath. Alcohol or nicotine on the breath may be noted. A sweet 'pear drops' smell may indicate ketosis, which is seen in starvation and diabetic ketoacidosis. A faecal smell on the breath can be noted in gastrointestinal obstruction (including constipation) and hepatic foetor is a musty smell associated with severe liver disease.

Neck

The symmetry of the neck should be observed. Are there any lumps or swellings? Lymphadenopathy in response to an upper respiratory tract infection is the most common cause of neck lumps. Swelling of the neck and face may indicate a parotid or submaxillary gland enlargement due to infection or duct stones. Or, as with any swelling or mass, it could be due to a tumour. Obvious masses in the neck such as goitre can be easily observed.

Are there any scars on the neck (either traumatic or from surgery such as a thyroidectomy), any skin lesions or radiotherapy skin changes? Are there any pulsations in the neck at the right-hand side, indicating a raised jugular venous pulse (JVP) in cardiovascular disease? Is the patient's voice hoarse; and if so, how long has the voice been hoarse? One of the most common causes is acute laryngitis, associated with upper respiratory tract infections such as the common cold or over-use of the voice following shouting or screaming. The former usually settles within 2 weeks and the latter within a week. Hoarseness persisting for more than 3 weeks could be due to age-related changes to the vocal cords or irritation caused by smoking or other irritants (such as acid reflux) or a sign of laryngeal cancer.

Hands

The patient's hands should be held and felt for temperature. If they are cold to the touch, this may indicate peripheral vascular disease or low cardiac output states such as shock. If, in addition to being cold, they feel moist and clammy, this may give further concern that the patient is presenting in a shocked state. Cold and clammy hands can also be found in states such as hypoglycaemia. Hands that feel inappropriately warm may be suggestive of a hyperactive thyroid disorder.

The patient's hands should be turned palms up and assessed for colour. Palmar erythema is excessive redness of the palm. This is perfectly normal in pregnancy but can also be seen in chronic liver disease. Nicotine staining of the fingers will be found in cigarette smokers. The patient's fingernails should next be checked; blue-tinged nails or peripheral cyanosis is caused by low oxygen saturations in tissues near the skin surface, as seen in a number of respiratory and cardiac conditions including circulatory conditions such as Raynaud's phenomenon.

Concave (spoon) nails (koilonychia) can be seen in iron-deficiency anaemia. Splinter haemorrhages are seen most frequently following trauma to the nail bed but can (in certain cases) be indicative of bacterial endocarditis. Clubbing of the nails, where there is loss of the angle at the base of the nail, is seen in a range of chronic cardiac, respiratory and gastrointestinal disorders. This can be tested for by asking the patient to place the nail beds of two opposing fingers together (say the index fingers of each hand). It should be possible to see a small diamond shape between the two nail beds. If the diamond is not present, this is a positive Schamroth's sign and finger clubbing is present. This may be idiopathic but is usually indicative of a number of different system disorders (respiratory, cardiovascular, gastrointestinal or dermatological).

Determining capillary refill time is a useful way of assessing a patient's peripheral circulation. One of the patient's fingers should be taken between the assessor's index finger and thumb and pressure should be gently applied on the nail bed until it blanches, then release the pressure and count the time it takes for the normal pink colour to return. If this time is longer than 2 seconds, this is an indicator of reduced peripheral blood flow which can be seen in respiratory distress, shock and other states where the sympathetic arm of the autonomic nervous system has been activated.

Symmetrical swelling of the joints of the hand may be seen in rheumatoid arthritis, whereas asymmetrical swelling is more indicative of osteoarthritis. The patient should be asked to extend their hand, palm-down. A fine tremor could be idiopathic but may also be a sign of a hepatic or neurological disorder. Xanthomata are the same fatty yellow deposits as in xanthelasma, which can grow in the tendons of the hands and feet and can be associated with high levels of cholesterol and triglyceride but can occur in the absence of hypercholesterolaemia.

Symptomology tips

- Loss of appetite is a characteristic of many illnesses such as infections and is short term. Persistent anorexia is a feature of more significant disease.
- Unintentional weight loss (that is, weight loss with no change in diet or exercise) is a sign of serious disease such as malignancy.

- New onset night sweats may be suggestive of serious disease, unless associated with endocrine conditions such as diabetes and hyperthyroidism or other changes such as the menopause.
- Respiratory symptoms may be caused by heart disease.
- Anaemia can cause dyspnoea.
- Rheumatoid arthritis and other connective tissue diseases may cause respiratory symptoms.
- Chronic cough can be caused by gastro-oesophageal reflux.
- Neuromuscular diseases may cause respiratory symptoms, particularly dyspnoea.

Measuring vital signs

Vital sign measurement is fundamental to physical examination, as vital signs provide a holistic overview of the body's state of health, as well as revealing serious medical emergency states. It might appear elementary but practitioners should ensure there is a clock or watch with a second hand available or use the stop watch on a mobile phone. In an emergency situation, a phone will not be appropriate or safe; a reliable, easily accessible timepiece is needed if assessing vital signs is likely to be a regular occurrence.

Pulse

The pulse is the expansion of an artery with each heart contraction, felt where an artery passes over a solid structure such as bone or cartilage. Pulses are felt in the carotid, brachial, radial femoral or popliteal area. The radial pulse is the most commonly used and easily located pulse. To measure it, the patient's arm should be in a comfortable position and the pulse is situated at the posterior wrist below the base of the thumb.

To take the radial pulse, two to three fingertips of the dominant hand are placed just below the thumb side of the palm. A pulsation will be felt; the key is to practise the pressure necessary to palpate the pulse. If the pressure is too light, the pulse will not be felt; while too much pressure may obstruct palpable blood flow. The rate should be counted for a minute. When the practitioner is competent, the pulse can be counted for 30 seconds or 15 seconds and multiplied by 2 or 4 respectively.

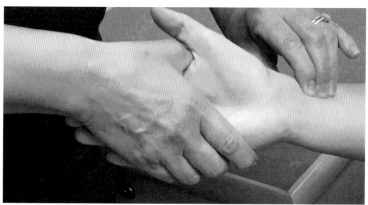

Figure 3.1: Taking the radial pulse

In addition to the rate of the pulse, it is also important to assess its rhythm and regularity and this can only be judged by a full minute measurement (see Table 3.1).

- A normal pulse rate for a healthy adult, after a period of rest, is between 60 and 80 beats per minute (bpm)
- A tachycardia is defined as a pulse rate in excess of 100 bpm
- A bradycardia is defined as a pulse rate less than 60 bpm
- A lower heart rate at rest can be due to more efficient heart function and superior cardiovascular fitness. For example, an athlete might have a normal resting heart rate closer to 40–50 beats a minute.

Table 3.1

Rhythm/regularity and clinical correlation	
Irregularly irregular (a pulse spaced erratically with no discernible pattern)	atrial fibrillation (or multiple ectopics)
Regularly irregular (a pulse where there is irregularity in a regular pattern)	2nd degree heart block
Water hammer pulse (strong radial pulse that taps the fingers on lifting of the patient's arm; indicates wide pulse pressure of aortic regurgitation)	aortic regurgitation
Bounding pulse (a strong pulse)	CO_2 retention, liver failure or sepsis
Small volume thready pulse (a weakly felt pulse)	shock
Radio-radial delay (a delay felt between the radial pulse in one wrist when taking the pulse simultaneously in each wrist)	can suggest coarctation or dissection of the aorta

Respiration

Biologically, respiration is the chemical process of breaking down glucose to release energy, for which oxygen is required. In the context of measuring vital signs, respiration is the process of breathing: inhalation and exhalation of air. In the strictest sense it is ventilation. Normal ventilation is an automatic, smooth and effortless process of inspiratory expansion and expiratory contraction of the chest with a fairly constant rate and rhythm. When in a resting state, the diaphragm is the main muscle of breathing, with some minor external intercostal action. The accessory muscles of inspiration, (the sternocleidomastoid and scalenes) and expiration (the internal intercostal and the abdominals) are employed during exercise but not when in a resting state. Clearly, if these accessory muscles are engaged when at rest there is increased respiratory effort which is not normal.

When observing patients' respiration rate, this should be done discreetly, as the automatic rhythm may be altered or controlled when the patient becomes aware that their breathing is being watched. One way of doing this is to continue to appear to be taking the pulse while discreetly starting to observe and count each respiration – that is, every rise (inspiration) and fall (expiration) of the chest. Each respiration should be counted for 60 seconds. If the patient's breathing is not discernible at rest, use a stethoscope to listen to the respirations over the tracheal/bronchial area. When the practitioner is competent, the respiratory rate can be counted for 30 seconds or 15 seconds and multiplied by 2 or 4 respectively.

Another important part of the respiratory assessment is the rhythm, regularity, depth and effort of breathing, which can also only be judged by a full minute measurement (see Table 3.2).

- The normal respiratory rate for a healthy adult, after a period of rest, is between 12 and 20 breaths per minute
- Tachypnoea is defined as a respiratory rate in excess of 25
- Bradypnoea is defined as a respiratory rate less than 11.

For this respiratory domain, all the additional signs and symptoms noted in the general assessment section of this chapter should be included.

Table 3.2

Rhythm/regularity/depth/effort of breathing and clinical correlation	
Orthopnoea/dyspnoea	pulmonary or cardiac impairment
Prolonged expiratory phase	chronic obstructive pulmonary disease (COPD) and asthma
Audible wheeze	acute asthma exacerbation, COPD (happy wheezer, pink puffer)
Intercostal retraction and tracheal/xiphisternum tugs (in-drawing recession at the tracheal notch/xiphisternum and intercostal spaces of the ribs)	severe restriction
Use of accessory muscles (sternomastoids, abdominals)	severe restriction
Cyanosis	severe restriction
Inspiratory stridor	interstitial oedema
Expiratory stridor	asthma and COPD
Irregular, fast and slow, deep and shallow, periods of apnoea (Cheyne-Stokes breathing)	heart failure, stroke, terminal/dying patients
Deep, rapid, laboured (Kussmaul's breathing)	late stage metabolic disorders, diabetic ketoacidosis

Temperature

In general practice settings, the tympanic thermometer (infrared in-ear thermometer [IRET]) is the most commonly used device for temperature measurement.

In hospital settings the temporal artery thermometer (TAT) is more commonly used. Both devices are hand-held. The IRET has a probe which is inserted into the ear canal and measures a combination of temperatures between the tympanic membrane and the external auditory meatus (EAM) to calculate a core temperature. The TAT is held over the forehead and senses infrared emissions radiating from the skin (Geijer *et al.* 2016).

The procedure for using the IRET is to remove the probe unit from its container and attach a probe cover to the IRET probe. The helix of the patient's ear should be pulled upward and back. The probe is then inserted into the ear canal, angling forward in line with the patient's mid cheek. The start button is depressed until the temperature reading is displayed on the digital unit (usually 2 seconds), the IRET is removed and the probe cover is disposed of; the temperature is recorded.

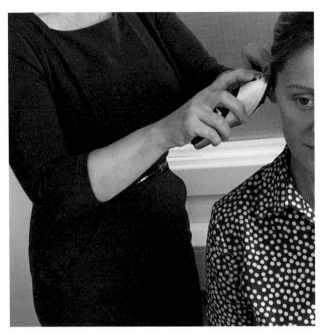

Figure 3.2: Taking a patient's temperature using an infrared in-ear thermometer

The procedure for using the TAT is first to clean the probe with an alcohol wipe and then ensure any hair is brushed aside if it is covering the patient's forehead or ear. The probe is placed flush on the centre of the forehead. The start button is depressed until the temperature reading is displayed on the digital unit. The probe is slowly slid midline across the forehead to the hairline across the temple, not down the side of the face. The probe should then be lifted from the forehead and run along the neck, just behind the ear lobe. The button can then be released, read and the temperature recorded. Finally, the probe is cleaned with an alcohol wipe.

Normal adult temperature is between 36.5 and 37.2°C. Temperatures ≤35.0°C and ≥39.1°C are considered red flag vital signs; 38.1–39.0°C is classified as amber and the patient needs close monitoring.

Oxygen saturations

Blood pumped from the heart is rich in oxygen (95–99% saturated) and the blood pumped back to the heart is low in oxygen (65–70%). All body cells demand oxygen in order to function. If oxygen delivery to the body cells falls below what is demanded, the tissues extract more oxygen from the haemoglobin and the saturation of the blood gases falls. All cells are dependent on an adequate, constant supply of oxygen, as they are unable to store it. The oxygen supply depends on an intact respiratory and cardiovascular function, which is limited by other factors such as peripheral shut-down. A reduction in oxygen can lead to organ dysfunction and death.

Pulse oximetry is a simple and non-invasive technique that is used to measure blood oxygenation (the percentage of haemoglobin that is oxygen-saturated). Probes are usually attached to the finger but can be attached to a toe.

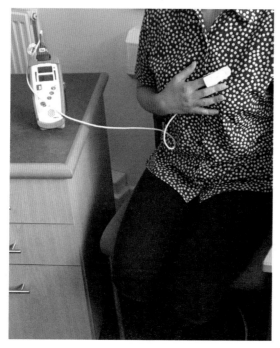

Figure 3.3: Using pulse oximetry to measure blood oxygenation

False readings may occur if there is anything that absorbs light, such as dried blood or nail polish. The patient's digit must be fully inserted into the probe. Appropriately sized probes should be used for children and infants. The hand should be placed on the chest at heart level to minimise motion artefact. Ideally, resting readings should be taken for at least 5 minutes. Poor pulse oximeter readings can be due to cold extremities – for example, the patient's hands could be cold from travelling to the surgery or hospital on a particularly chilly day. Normal oxygen saturation in adults is 95% and above.

Blood pressure

Blood pressure (BP) is a measure of the force the heart exerts to circulate blood and also the pressure of the circulating blood on the inner walls of blood vessels. Cardiac output, blood volume, peripheral resistance and arterial elasticity or stiffness vary depending on activity or inactivity, emotional state and relative health and/or disease state. The BP is expressed as systolic and diastolic blood pressure and is stated in terms of millimetres of mercury (mmHg). Systolic pressure is the maximum blood pressure exerted during contraction of the ventricles; the diastolic pressure is the minimum pressure, when the heart is relaxed prior to the next contraction.

The following description of BP measurement technique is based on the British Hypertension Society (BHS) recommendations (NICE 2016). Automated devices are now commonly used in most healthcare settings. However, many automated devices may not measure blood pressure accurately if there is pulse irregularity (due to atrial fibrillation, for example). If pulse irregularity is present, the BP should be measured manually, using direct auscultation over the brachial artery.

Manual BP measurement, using an aneroid sphygmomanometer and a stethoscope, is a complex procedure which takes many hours of practice to master. Manual sphygmomanometry is based on a technique introduced by Scipione Riva-Rocci in 1896 and modified by Nikolai Korotkoff in 1905. The tapping sounds heard through the stethoscope are called Korotkoff sounds. The systolic blood pressure is taken to be the pressure at which the first Korotkoff sound is first heard and the diastolic blood pressure is the pressure at which the fifth Korotkoff sound is heard – that is, the last sound before the tapping disappears.

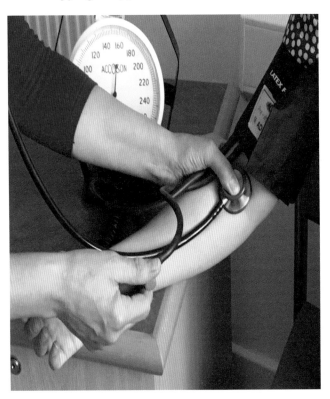

Figure 3.4: Taking a patient's blood pressure

Before taking the patient's BP, the procedure is briefly outlined. In particular, the patient should be warned about the minor discomfort caused by inflation and deflation of the cuff and that the measurement may be repeated several times. The patient should be asked to uncover their upper arm by rolling up the sleeve. If the sleeve is tight and therefore restrictive, the patient should be asked to remove their arm from the sleeve completely. The appropriate size cuff should be selected, as per Table 3.3. Alcohol wipes are used to clean the cuff that will be in contact with the patient's skin and also the stethoscope diaphragm and earpieces. The patient is positioned, with their arm extended and supported in line with the heart. The brachial pulse is located by palpation and then the cuff is wrapped around the patient's upper arm, ensuring that the centre of the cuff bladder is positioned over the line of the brachial artery. The lower edge of the cuff should be 2–3cm above the antecubital fossa and should be well secured and sit firmly on the arm.

The radial or brachial pulse is palpated and the cuff inflated until the pulse is no longer palpable (the estimated systolic). The cuff is then rapidly deflated and the estimated systolic noted. The diaphragm of the stethoscope is placed over the brachial artery and secured by placing a thumb over the bell of the stethoscope and wrapping the other fingers around the back of the patient's elbow holding their arm extended. The cuff is re-inflated to 20–30mmHg over the estimated systolic. The cuff is then deflated at 2–3mmHg per second. The first two consecutive Korotkoff sounds of the systolic blood pressure should be noted, as should the disappearance of Korotkoff sounds as representing the diastolic blood pressure. The BP results should be written down immediately. The cuff is then removed, cleaned with an alcohol wipe and the patient left comfortable.

When considering a diagnosis of hypertension, the BP should be measured in both arms. If there is a difference of 10–20mmHg, subsequent readings should be taken in the arm with the higher reading. A diagnosis of hypertension should not be made on clinic readings alone. In addition, 24-hour ambulatory BP monitoring (ABPM) daytime average or home BP monitoring (HBPM) average blood pressure readings should be obtained.

British Hypertension Society (BHS) reference ranges:

Stage 1 hypertension – clinic blood pressure is 140/90mmHg or higher and subsequent ABPM daytime average or HBPM average blood pressure is 135/85mmHg or higher

Stage 2 hypertension – clinic blood pressure is 160/100mmHg or higher and subsequent ABPM daytime average or HBPM average blood pressure is 150/95mmHg or higher

Severe hypertension – clinic systolic blood pressure is 180mmHg or higher or clinic diastolic blood pressure is 110mmHg or higher.

Table 3.3

Blood pressure cuff sizes for aneroid sphygmomanometer, semi-automatic and ambulatory monitors		
Indication bladder	Width/length (cm)	Arm circumference (cm)
Small adult/child	12 x 18	<23
Standard adult	12 x 26	<33
Large adult	12 x 40	<50
Adult thigh cuff	20 x 42	<53

Identifying and monitoring the deteriorating patient

In any healthcare setting, prescribers and other healthcare professionals need to be able to spot a deteriorating patient. Detailed below is the National Early Warning Score (NEWS) 2 (RCP 2017), which has now received formal endorsement from NHS and NHS Improvement to be used for identifying acutely ill patients (including those with sepsis) in the UK. The score is used to aid early recognition of a deteriorating patient, and it is based on physiological parameters. An aggregated score is calculated, and an escalation pathway is activated for specific scores.

(NEWS) 2 has a Track and Trigger approach; observations are taken by staff 12-hourly as a minimum and increased if there are signs of deterioration, staff are trained to understand the clinical relevance of the vital signs. The escalation pathway outlines actions required for timely review, ensuring appropriate interventions.

Who is at risk?

- Anyone in hospital
- Those with co-existing disease
- All emergency admissions
- Elderly people
- Those with specific acute illness (e.g. sepsis, pancreatitis)
- Those with an altered level of consciousness
- Those with major haemorrhage.

Possible causes of deterioration

- Sepsis
- Hospital-acquired infections
- Chronic disease process
- Comorbidities
- Unavoidable complications
- Failure to manage complications
- Reaching palliative/end of life stage.

Which vital signs need checking?

- Respiratory rate
- Oxygen saturations
- Pulse
- Systolic BP
- AVPU (Alert, Voice, Pain, Unresponsive)
- Temperature
- (Urine output is not in the scoring system but is an important marker of acute deterioration).

Respiratory rate – this is the most sensitive indicator of potential deterioration, with rising rates often being an early sign. As detailed earlier, this is noted in conjunction with other evidence (such as use of accessory muscles, increased work of breathing, struggling to speak in full sentences, exhaustion, and the colour of patient).

Oxygen saturations – be aware of appropriate 'target saturations' for individual patients (those with COPD, for example, have target saturations of between 88% and 95%). All acutely unwell patients should receive supplementary oxygen, which should be titrated according to their readings. NICE consider oxygen a drug.

Pulse rate – in patients who are at risk of deterioration, the pulse should be taken manually for 1 minute, noting the rate, volume and regularity as described earlier. Abnormal findings need investigating and should be followed with an electrocardiogram (ECG).

Blood pressure – organs are very dependent on adequate pressures to ensure perfusion. Adequate BP is essential for delivery of oxygen and nutrients to the rest of the body. The pressure in the arteries is carefully regulated by the body. If it drops, immediate circulatory changes occur:

- The heart rate increases
- Blood vessels constrict so the BP may remain adequate
- Capillary refill time decreases
- Urine output decreases.

Blood pressure alteration is a late sign of deterioration – patients will compensate (especially the young). What is normal for the patient should be noted.

The AVPU scale is a system to measure and record a patient's level of consciousness. It is a mnemonic for Alert, Voice, Pain, Unresponsive:

ALERT: The patient is responsive to any stimuli, though they may be disorientated and confused. There is spontaneous eye opening in response to voice or physical stimuli. There is bodily motor function.

VOICE: The patient responds when spoken to, either by eye movement or verbally by a moan or grunt or physical movement such as movement of a limb.

PAIN: The patient responds to peripheral pain stimulus, such as pinching the ear or pressing into the bed of a fingernail, or central stimuli such as a sternal rub. A fully conscious patient will respond to the pain and push it away, whereas a patient who is not alert and not responding to voice stimuli may only manifest involuntary flexion or extension of a limb.

UNRESPONSIVE: Sometimes described as unconscious, this outcome is noted if the patient does not have any Eye, Voice or Motor response to voice or pain.

The Resuscitation Council describes what to do if a patient has an AVPU response of P or U (Resuscitation Council UK 2015).

Temperature: This can have a significant effect on the patient's condition. High or low temperature can indicate sepsis; low can be as important as high. Significant warming can cause vasodilatation. In at-risk patients with pyrexia of > 38°C, consider arranging for blood cultures.

Urine output: This is a sensitive indicator of hydration status and, due to high demand for blood supply to the kidneys, urine output is also a useful indicator of cardiovascular status.

- Normal output should be 0.5ml/kg/hr.
- Fluid balance should be monitored in at-risk patients.
- In acute kidney injury, urine output decreases, toxic waste increases and the patient needs urgent attention.

Chain of safety and escalation pathway

Measure vital signs and document

↓

Recognise deterioration

↓

Communicate appropriately

↓

Respond efficiently and reassess

SBAR (Situation, Background, Assessment, Recommendation) is a tool used to communicate critical information succinctly and briefly between healthcare practitioners. It is very straightforward to use (DH 2011).

SITUATION: Briefly describe the situation. Give a succinct overview.
The assessor gives their name and why they are calling.

BACKGROUND: Briefly state pertinent history.
Describe the patient's condition now and what the norm is for this patient.

ASSESSMENT: Summarise the facts. What could be going on?
Suggest a possible reason for deterioration.

RECOMMENDATION: What is being asked for? What needs to happen next?
Come and see the patient in x minutes or ask what to do next.

Summary

By becoming prescribers, pharmacists have an opportunity to expand their role and take on all aspects of the patient journey, from diagnosis to prescribing, advice and follow-up. This chapter has presented a brief overview of physical examination skills, clinical assessment and general common physical signs of ill health and red flags. If a pharmacist is in a prescribing role where they will be expected to regularly examine patients, it is strongly recommended that they undertake at least a further module in clinical reasoning and physical assessment in order to fulfil such a specialist role.

References

Department of Health (DH) (2011). *NHS Improvements. SBAR communication tool – situation, background, assessment, recommendation.* https://improvement.nhs.uk/resources/sbar-communication-tool (last accessed 19.5.2019).

Geijer, H., Udumyan, R., Lohse G. & Nilsagård Y. (2016). Temperature measurements with a temporal scanner: systematic review and meta-analysis. *British Medical Journal Open.* **6** (3).

General Pharmaceutical Council (GPhC) (Undated). *Pharmacist independent prescribing programme – learning outcomes and indicative content.* https://www.pharmacyregulation.org/sites/default/files/pharmacist_independent_prescribing_-_learning_outcomes_and_indicative_content.pdf (last accessed 28.5.2019).

General Pharmaceutical Council (GPhC) (2011). https://www.pharmacyregulation.org/sites/default/files/document/gphc_future_pharmacists_may_2011.pdf (last accessed 17.5.2019).

General Pharmaceutical Council (GPhC) (2012). *Guidance on maintaining clear sexual boundaries.* https://www.pharmacyregulation.org/sites/default/files/gphc_guidance_on_sexual_boundaries_14.pdf (last accessed 19.5.2019).

General Pharmaceutical Council (GPhC) (2016). *Prescribers Survey Report.* https://www.pharmacyregulation.org/sites/default/files/gphc_prescribers_survey_report.pdf (last accessed 14.5.2019).

National Institute for Health and Care Excellence (NICE) (2016). *Hypertension in adults: diagnosis and management. Clinical guideline [CG127]* Published August 2011; last updated November 2016. https://www.nice.org.uk/guidance/cg127 (last accessed 19.5.2019).

National Institute for Health and Care Excellence (NICE) (2017). *Healthcare-associated infections: prevention and control in primary and community care. Clinical guideline [CG139].* Published March 2012; last updated February 2017. https://www.nice.org.uk/guidance/cg139 (last accessed 19.5.2019).

McCallum, L. & Higgins, D. (2012) Measuring body temperature. *Nursing Times.* **108**(45), 20–22.

Resuscitation Council UK (2015). *Guidelines and guidance: The ABCDE approach.* https://www.resus.org.uk/resuscitation-guidelines/abcde-approach (last accessed 19.5.2019).

Royal College of Physicians (RCP) (2017). *National Early Warning Score (NEWS) 2. Standardising the assessment of acute illness in the NHS.* https://www.rcplondon.ac.uk/projects/outputs/national-early-warning-score-news-2 (last accessed 19.5.2019).

Royal Pharmaceutical Society (RPS) (2016). *A Competency Framework for All Prescribers.* London: RPS. https://www.rpharms.com/Portals/0/RPS%20document%20library/Open%20access/Professional%20standards/Prescribing%20competency%20framework/prescribing-competency-framework.pdf (last accessed 14.5.2019).

4

Patient partnership and prescribing

Rani Khatib, Janet Holt, Catherine Gill
and Barry Strickland-Hodge

Chapter overview

In this chapter a number of issues around the patient–prescriber partnership will be considered. The areas to be covered are:

- Medicines optimisation, including adherence to therapy and issues of polypharmacy and multi-morbidity
- Cultural and religious considerations in prescribing
- Ethical considerations
- Public health issues.

In the *Competency Framework for All Prescribers* (RPS 2016; see Appendix), the patient partnership is a central theme in a number of competencies – for example, Competency 3 ('Reach a shared decision') and in particular statement 3.2 'identifying and respecting the patient in relation to diversity, values, beliefs and expectations about their health'. Competency 5 ('Provide information') is also particularly relevant to the patient–prescriber partnership.

Medicines optimisation

The most common intervention in healthcare is the prescribing of medicines to alleviate disease, manage long-term conditions and prevent illness. The management of medicines in healthcare systems is crucial, but it is more important that patients derive the best-quality outcomes from their medicines. The National Institute for Health and Care Excellence defines medicines optimisation as 'a person-centred approach to safe and effective medicines use, to ensure people obtain the best possible outcomes from their medicines' (NICE 2015).

Accumulating evidence relating to the use of medicines highlighted a need to shift the balance from how the system manages medicines to how the patient manages their medicines. Average non-adherence to prescribed medicines among patients with long-term conditions is estimated to be 33–50%. Ten days after starting a new medicine, 30% of patients are not taking them as prescribed (Barber *et al.* 2004). This can lead to negative consequences for the patient, including worsening of the condition, increased comorbidities, admission to hospital and potentially death. Impacts on the the healthcare system include increased costs and medicines waste. It is estimated that NHS primary and community care prescription medicines waste costs £300 million a year (Trueman *et al.* 2010).

In the Competency Framework, Competency 3, statement 3.4, is 'routinely assesses adherence in a non-judgemental way and understands the different reasons non-adherence can occur (intentional or non-intentional) and how best to support patients/carers'. Similarly, Competency 1, statement 1.7, says 'reviews adherence to and effectiveness of current medicines'. (RPS 2016; see Appendix).

With an ageing population comes the challenge of multi-morbidity, defined as the presence of two or more long-term conditions in one person. Multi-morbidity is associated with higher mortality, increased hospital admissions, and being prescribed multiple medicines (or polypharmacy), which increases the 'medicines burden' on patients. The King's Fund report on polypharmacy defined it as 'the concurrent use of multiple medications by one individual' and went on to identify the need for medicines optimisation to distinguish between appropriate polypharmacy with the potential to do good, and problematic polypharmacy with the potential to do harm – for example, through drug interactions and adverse drug reactions (Duerden, Avery & Payne 2013).

Multi-morbidity does not seem to be confined to the older population. In a Canadian study 93% of patients aged 45–64 had multi-morbidity, which in turn leads to polypharmacy (Fortin *et al.* 2005). In another report, ineffective or inappropriate use of medicines was associated with 5–8% of hospital admissions and 6.5% of admissions were a result of adverse effects of medicines (Pirmohamed *et al.* 2004).

Medicines optimisation constitutes a shift away from medicines management, a term used to encompass all systems, activities, behaviours and processes relating to the use of medicines by patients, and – more broadly – by the NHS. Medicines management tends to focus on systems – in other words, prescribing budgets, spending and costs. Medicines optimisation focuses on patients and how they use medicines to achieve better outcomes. Its success is measured in terms of improved patient experience, reduced referrals and unplanned admissions, reduced medicine waste, increased quality of care and improved outcomes.

Healthcare professionals are encouraged to adopt the Royal Pharmaceutical Society's four guiding principles for medicines optimisation:

- Aim to understand the patient's experience
- Ensure there is an evidence-based choice of medicines available
- Ensure medicines use is as safe as possible
- Make medicines optimisation part of routine practice (RPS 2013).

The approach should always be patient-centred. The effectiveness of medicines optimisation is measured by improved patient outcomes, as illustrated in Figure 4.1. While pharmacists can provide leadership and support for medicines optimisation, the Royal Pharmaceutical Society emphasises that the principles need to be followed by everyone involved in the patient's care pathway.

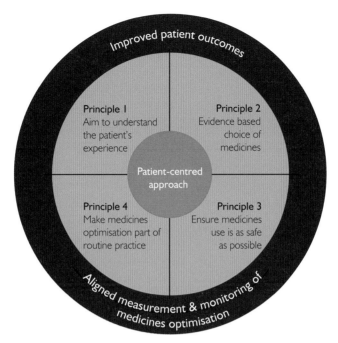

Figure 4.1: From Medicines Optimisation:
Helping patients to make the most of medicines (RPS 2013).
Diagram reproduced with the permission of the Royal Pharmaceutical Society.

NICE published a Quality Standard for Medicines Optimisation (QS120) in March 2016 to ensure that its guidance on medicines optimisation is better implemented. The standards highlight the high-priority areas for quality improvement alongside recommendations supporting measurement of this improvement. Table 4.1 lists the six quality statements (NICE 2016).

NICE quality statements for medicines optimisation

1. People are given the opportunity to be involved in making decisions about their medicines.
2. People who are prescribed medicines are given an explanation on how to identify and report medicines-related patient safety incidents.
3. Local health and social care providers monitor medicines-related patient safety incidents to inform their learning in the use of medicines.
4. People who are inpatients in an acute setting have a reconciled list of their medicines within 24 hours of admission.
5. People discharged from a care setting have a reconciled list of their medicines in their GP record within one week of the GP practice receiving the information, and before a prescription or new supply of medicines is issued.
6. Local healthcare providers identify people taking medicines who would benefit from a structured medication review.

The best possible outcomes from medicines use require an open dialogue with the patient and/or their carer about their health and beliefs about medicines, their preferred choice and their experience of using medicines. Doyle *et al.* (2013) emphasised that the patient experience is one of the three dimensions of quality in healthcare that should be considered collectively, alongside clinical effectiveness and patient safety.

Engaging with patients to understand their medicine-taking experience requires practitioners to apply the concept of shared decision-making, and provide clear patient-tailored information and respect for patient choices. This should help in improving adherence as patients are more likely to take ownership of their medicines and not feel 'judged' when they share their non-adherence behaviour (which they may otherwise be reluctant to disclose).

It is important to remember that patient experience also includes practical aspects of medicines use, such as accessing and taking medicines, repeat prescriptions, swallowing tablets or capsules, opening bottles, etc. Problems with any of these aspects should be explored and addressed.

The NICE Quality statement 1 (NICE 2016) emphasises the shared decision-making approach. It builds on the premise that decisions about medicines made jointly between the patient and the prescriber are likely to lead to better clinical outcomes and patient satisfaction. The choice made by the patient may include decisions not to take specific medicines.

After understanding the needs of the patients, the pharmacist prescriber should ensure that the medicines offered to the patient are the most appropriate clinical and cost-effective choices. This decision needs to be informed by the best available evidence base. Competency 7 ('Prescribe safely') and Competency 8 ('Prescribe professionally') includes this basic concept (RPS 2016; see Appendix).

The best sources of evidence-based recommendations are national and international guidelines such as those published by NICE. Currently, in the UK, NICE guidelines make recommendations about how healthcare professionals should care for people with specific conditions and which medicines should be offered, based on robust evidence and cost-effectiveness studies. In the absence of national or international guidelines, local formularies and peer-reviewed clinical evidence summaries or recommendations are a good alternative.

It is very important to remember that evidence-based choices should always be tailored to the individual needs of patients. NICE recommends a patient-centred approach when implementing guidelines, and also makes its guidance accessible to patients and has developed some patient decision aids (PDAs). Evidence-based guidelines are rarely produced in a format that supports shared decision-making. This means the prescriber needs to make an extra effort to ensure that patients are making an informed choice. This area of prescribing practice is included in Competency 5 ('Provide information') and the five elements of this competency are designed to help both the prescriber and the patient get the best from prescribed medicines (RPS 2016; see Appendix).

Implementing the NICE QS120 requires healthcare providers to collect evidence to show that patients are being given suitable information about the potential benefits and harms of using medicines. They also need to demonstrate that people's preferences and values regarding treatment options have been taken into account. Surveying patients and collecting their feedback is essential (GPhC 2016). The four elements of Competency 6 ('Monitor and review') cover these aspects (RPS 2016; see Appendix).

The Hippocratic Oath states 'Also I will, according to my ability and judgment, prescribe a regimen for the health of the sick; but I will utterly reject harm and mischief'; this is usually summed by the phrase 'First Do No Harm'.

While ensuring that patients get the best outcome from their medicines, every effort must be made to prevent harm. The safe use of medicines covers all aspects of medicines handling, from production to administering and monitoring. This is the responsibility of all professionals, healthcare organisations and patients. The safety aspect of taking medicines should be part of the discussion with patients and/or their carers. For example, Competency 3, statement 3.3, is 'explains the rationale behind and potential risks and benefits of management options in a way the patient/carer understands'. Similarly, Competency 7, 'Prescribe safely' (RPS 2016; see Appendix) deals with the safety aspects of medicines.

Healthcare organisations and professionals should ensure better reporting and prevention of safety incidents related to medicines. These incidents may include errors in prescribing, preparing, dispensing, administering, monitoring, providing advice on medicines and communications between healthcare professionals and different healthcare settings about patients' medicines. Reporting, and learning from, incidents related to patient safety has improved significantly in the last decade and this can be seen in local and national initiatives, such as the Medicines and Healthcare products Regulatory Agency (MHRA) patient safety alerts, the National Reporting and Learning System (NRLS) and the Yellow Card Scheme (MHRA). This is highlighted in NICE Quality Statement 3 (GPhC 2016) and in the *Competency Framework*, where statement 7.6 is 'reports prescribing errors, near misses and critical incidents and reviews practice to prevent recurrence' (RPS 2016; see Appendix).

The NICE Quality Statement 2 (GPhC 2016) expects healthcare professionals to encourage and empower patients to report incidents in order to make reporting and learning from medicines-related patient safety incidents more effective. This requires healthcare professionals to advise patients on how to identify and report medicines-related patient safety incidents when a prescription is written or dispensed, or at medication review. This should increase the number of incidents reported, and can aid patients' learning. The other aspect related to this Quality Statement is enabling the patient to reduce harm from adverse drug reactions by being able to identify them and know what to do about them (GPhC 2016). Competency Statement 5.2 includes 'gives the patient/carer clear, understandable and accessible information about their medicines (e.g. what it is for etc... how to use it, possible unwanted effects and how to report them, expected duration of treatment)' (RPS 2016; see Appendix).

As most medication errors seem to occur during transfer of care, NICE Quality Statements 4 and 5 stress the need for medicines reconciliation during these episodes (GPhC 2016). Medicines reconciliation ensures that any discrepancies and changes to medicines (including over-the-counter medicines and supplements) are identified. This not only reduces errors, but also ensures the accuracy, quality and relevance of the patient's management plan. Statement 4.13 of the *Competency Framework* is 'communicates information about medicines and what they are being used for when sharing or transferring prescribing responsibilities/information' (RPS 2016; see Appendix).

Medicines reviews, as in NICE Quality Statement 6, are also important in identifying the appropriateness, relevance and safety of medicines prescribed. This is particularly relevant to patients with long-term conditions, those with multi-morbidity and polypharmacy, and those being prescribed high-risk medicines (NICE 2016). For more on this, see also Chapters 5 and 6.

Medicines optimisation should be embedded within all clinical practice. Healthcare professionals should make every effort to ensure that getting the best outcomes from medicines is integrated as part of healthcare pathways and routinely carried out as part of patients' care. This requires discussion with patients and/or their carers and with other healthcare professionals, in the form of medicines reconciliation and regular review of a patient's medicines. A medicines review, as defined by NICE (2016), should be:

> a structured, critical examination of a person's medicines with the objective of reaching an agreement with the person about treatment, optimising the impact of medicines, minimising the number of medication-related problems, and reducing waste.

The medicines review could be conducted as a standalone service or as part of a clinical consultation with the patient. Depending on their specific needs and the complexity of their treatment, individual patients may need more in-depth medicines reviews carried out by specialist healthcare professionals such as pharmacists (NICE 2015).

In his report, Lord Carter made practical recommendations which embedded medicines optimisation in NHS hospitals. He identified a key role for pharmacists, as part of £5 billion of savings that can be made through better workforce and resource management. According to his report (Carter 2016, p. 7) Trusts should use at least 80% of their pharmacist resource for direct medicines optimisation activities, medicines governance and safety remits. Lord Carter considered the delivery of hospital pharmacy services, to be inseparable from the optimisation of medicines:

> In hospital pharmacy we know that the more time pharmacists spend on clinical services rather than infrastructure or back-office services, the more likely medicines use is optimised.

Summary of medicines optimisation

Medicines optimisation, as detailed in the Royal Pharmaceutical Society principles (RPS 2013) and the NICE (2015) guideline and quality statements, is a new approach and way of working that aims to maximise patient benefit from medicines and improve the quality and safety of medicines use. Medicines optimisation is patient-centred. It is based on understanding the patient experience when taking medicines and encouraging significant involvement of patients in decisions about their medicines to provide individualised healthcare that is tailored to the individual patient's needs.

Practical issues encountered with medicines and religious beliefs

Prescribers must take into account patients' beliefs (religious, cultural or other) and involve them in all aspects of the prescribing consultation (see also Chapter 2). Competency 3 ('Reach a shared decision') includes statement 3.2: 'identifies and respects the patient in relation to diversity, values, beliefs and expectations about their health and treatment with medicines' and statement 3.1: 'works with the patient/carers in partnership to make informed choices, agreeing a plan that respects patient preferences, including their right to refuse or limit treatment'. Other parts of Competency 3 are also relevant at this point (RPS 2016; see Appendix).

Patients may have personal reasons for not wanting to take suggested medication. One obvious reason would be real or perceived allergies. The patient's allergy status will be available via their medical notes, which should be confirmed with the patient at each consultation (see Chapter 2). This ensures the medical notes are kept up to date in case any new allergies or reactions arise.

In addition to their allergy status, patients may have preferences about the types of medicines they will or will not take. These preferences may be based on religious or cultural considerations. For example, the Muslim and Jewish populations are prohibited from consuming pork and may therefore want to avoid medicines that are derived from pigs. Prescribers must carefully consider these beliefs and include a discussion of potential treatments, where relevant, in the prescriber–patient consultation. Patients are much more likely to adhere to medicine recommendations if they are actively involved in the decision- making process and their beliefs are constructively taken into account.

How are these issues identified?

Many medicines and many different dosage forms contain animal derivatives. In 1995, the World Health Organisation participated in a seminar with the Islamic organisation for medical sciences in Kuwait on the topic 'The Judicially Prohibited and Impure Substances in Foodstuffs and Drugs' (WHO 1995). The seminar offered a number of recommendations, including a point on transformation (that is, when substances have been converted into something else with different characteristics). This can potentially change the substance into a pure form, from an impure form, for those from particular religious groups. A statement was then given: 'The gelatin formed as a result of the transformation of the bones, skin and tendons of a judicially impure animal is pure and it is judicially permissible to eat it' (WHO 1995).

The publication was disseminated in 2001 and includes a nine-point statement. Regarding medication of animal origin (such as some forms of insulin), necessities overrule prohibitions. There is a basic rule which states that all things are lawful unless specifically prohibited. For instance, for Muslims, although wine and other intoxicants may be unlawful there is no objection from the point of view of Sharia law to using alcohol as an antiseptic or a disinfectant. A discussion is warranted with patients with diabetes explaining that the use of animal-derived insulin is permissible because of necessity if there are no alternatives.

However, it would be prudent to avoid animal derivatives for insulin and other medicines wherever possible. Something that is 'unclean' may become 'clean' and permissible by the transformation of the original substance. However, pig fat used in an ointment remains unclean as its properties have not changed (WHO 1995).

For Jewish patients, Jewish law permits the consumption of porcine and other non-kosher materials in a non-edible form in the case of illness (as in injections and parenteral administration of such products). For example, injectable porcine-derived insulin is permitted if there is no alternative. In contrast, any food or dietary additive or medicine that is to be swallowed must contain only kosher ingredients. Other areas of consideration may include lactose, which is contained in many tablets, as Jewish laws prohibit the consumption of milk and meat together. While such tablets may be permitted as the lactose is not 'edible', more thought should be given when considering lactulose. Dietary requirements for many religious groups may change depending on the time of year; for instance, the use of wheat starch during Passover should be further researched.

Informed consent must be obtained from all patients by all prescribers. Questions that could be asked include, 'has the patient been made aware that their treatment may include medicines derived from animals?' 'If not, why is this?' The prescriber should become aware of their patients' religious beliefs or preferences. As discussed in Chapter 2, effective communication is important for the role of a pharmacist, and it is essential in a prescribing role. There may be particular questions from Jewish patients, Muslims, Hindus, Jehovah's Witnesses and others, so a knowledge of patients' religious beliefs is important for prescribers.

The key to a good and effective prescriber–patient relationship is to be aware of what alternatives may be available. There has been a move from biologically sourced to synthetic forms of drugs. However, the animal origin of any drug treatment should form part of any clinical decision-making. To use insulin as an example, the earliest formulations were directly extracted from the pancreas of cows and pigs, whereas current formulations include recombinant human insulin or synthetically derived insulin analogues.

Another example involves low molecular weight heparins, which are routinely used in the hospital setting for venous thromboembolism prevention. Low molecular weight heparins may be derived from pigs but there is one synthetic preparation available – fondaparinux. Patients who have specific requirements or preferences should be offered a choice, if a choice exists. If it does not, this discussion needs to form part of the consultation. For information about the animal origin of medicines, use the online resource www.medicines.org.uk (Datapharm 2019) and view the Summary of Product Characteristics or contact the manufacturer directly. Not all medicines are covered but the majority are.

In 2013, the Department of Health in Queensland, Australia, produced a guideline on medicines of animal origin. This lists several religious groups who may object to certain medicines or particular dosage forms. Also, in the guide is a list of medicines incorporating porcine, bovine and other derivatives which may potentially be inappropriate for certain patient groups or individuals (Queensland DOH 2013).

The Australian Guideline includes a table which looks at religious restrictions for seven religions, from Buddhism to Sikhism. It also has information relating to medicinal products and which animal they are derived from, and which products may contain eggs or other potentially restricted excipients (inactive substances).

For prescribers, knowledge of a patient's preferences in relation to animal-derived medications will help inform the decision-making process when selecting a medication. This may ultimately help to ensure adherence by patients and reduce costs associated with non-adherence and waste.

Questions may also be asked about drugs of animal origin for vegetarians or vegans. For example, as the UK-based Vegan Society observes (Chew 2013):

> …we live in an imperfect world. … In The Vegan Society's Memorandum of Association, veganism is used to denote a philosophy and way of living which seeks to exclude, as far as possible and practicable, all forms of exploitation of, and cruelty to, animals. You yourself know best what your own particular situation is, what efforts you can make and what possible and practicable means for you.

Ethical considerations relating to the supply and administration of medicines

Prescribing governance is the second domain in the *Competency Framework for All Prescribers* and includes Competencies 7–10. Competency 7 ('Prescribe safely'), statement 7.2, deals with working within a scope of practice; and statement 7.6 covers reporting prescribing errors, near misses, critical incidents and reviewing practice to prevent recurrence. Legal and regulatory frameworks are covered in Competency 8 ('Prescribes professionally'), statement 8.3 'knows and works within legal and regulatory frameworks affecting prescribing practice' (RPS 2016; see Appendix).

Ethical practice

Ethical practice is about acting morally or, to put it another way, doing the right thing. In contemporary value-based healthcare, practitioners often face moral dilemmas and then have to make decisions on how to act to do the right thing (Benson *et al.* 2009). Beauchamp and Childress (2013) explain that moral dilemmas occur when there are at least two alternative but incompatible courses of action and the person has to make a choice about what to do.

Moral dilemmas

When faced with a moral dilemma, not only does a choice have to be made as to which path to follow, but the decision also needs to be justified. Decisions made when facing moral dilemmas in professional practice (including prescribing) may have to be justified to a range of people such as colleagues, line managers, service users and professional bodies. There are a number of ways in which decisions may be justified and, for most people, this will start with an appeal to conscience. However, conscience can be an ambiguous concept, which gives rise to conflict, as it is quite possible for two people to follow their individual consciences and hold diametrically opposed views on the right course of action. We may therefore understand that our conscience is telling us to act in a certain way but determining whether that is indeed the correct way to act is a different matter (Gillon 1985).

Hearings before the General Pharmaceutical Council's Fitness to Practice Committee will determine whether a pharmacist's conduct is in accordance with the *Standards for pharmacy professionals* (GPhC 2017b). The role of the panel is to measure practitioners' conduct against the prescribed standards rather than make moral judgements. The *Standards for pharmacy professionals document*, while detailing the ways in which pharmacists should behave, offers no moral advice on how to deal with particular ethical conflicts when they arise.

Many of the ethical dilemmas that arise in practice leave practitioners facing moral choices that will not be addressed either in a court of law or by a regulatory body. If appealing to conscience is not a reliable method, we must look to other ways of addressing moral issues such as referring to ethical theory. According to Bennett (2010), studying ethics becomes a more pressing interest when the need to make correct moral or value judgements, such as those encountered in practice, is taken seriously. In making such judgements, we should first try to clearly express what the issues are. This will enable us to discuss them openly, reflect on them and evaluate them. Only then will we be in a position to decide on our moral position and be prepared to defend a particular course of action.

Competency 9 ('Improve prescribing practice') contains statement 9.1: 'reflects on own and others' prescribing practice, and acts upon feedback and discussion'. In Competency 8 ('Prescribe professionally'), statement 8.2 is 'accepts personal responsibility for prescribing and understands the legal and ethical implications' (RPS 2016; see Appendix).

Ethical theory

There are several ethical theories that prescribers should consider. In addition to classical theories, one approach that has proven popular among healthcare practitioners is that proposed by two American philosophers, Beauchamp and Childress, in their book *Principles of Biomedical Ethics* (Beauchamp & Childress 2013). First published in 1977, the theory focuses on four moral principles, namely: respect for autonomy; non-maleficence; beneficence; and justice, which the authors explain is a framework of norms pivotal in healthcare ethics. The theory is therefore about how the principles relate to, and can be used to guide, the prescriber.

Respect for autonomy

The notion of 'self-rule' underpins a belief that people are capable of making their own decisions, something of importance in the British healthcare system and a feature running through the NHS Constitution (DH 2015). It is also the foundation of the law pertaining to consent. An autonomous person should therefore be free to make decisions, free from controlling influences and in accordance with their own choices.

As mentioned earlier, Competency 3 ('Reach a shared decision') includes statement 3.1: 'works with the patient/carers in partnership to make informed choices, agreeing a plan that respects patient preferences including their right to refuse or limit treatment' (RPS 2016; see

Appendix). But there are circumstances which limit autonomy – for example, if there are defects in a person's control, or reasoning; defects in the information they have available; or instability in their decision-making because they keep changing their mind (Harris 1985). If none of these issues are present, then, in order to act morally, the practitioner should acknowledge and respect the view that a person has 'a right to hold views, make choices and take actions based on their values and beliefs' (Beauchamp & Childress, 2013, p. 106).

Non-maleficence and beneficence

While Beauchamp and Childress identify these as two separate principles, it is helpful for us to consider them together. Non-maleficence, the principle of avoiding harm, has a long history in healthcare and was first associated with the Hippocratic Oath (mentioned earlier), while the principle of beneficence is concerned with acting for the benefit of others. In many circumstances, a duty to avoid harm may be more important than an obligation to help others. Deciding whether an action is beneficial or harmful is the key ethical issue any prescriber is likely to face – for instance, dealing with a patient who is insisting on having antibiotics prescribed for what is suspected to be a viral infection.

Justice

The concept of justice implies fairness, in the sense of giving people what they deserve or are entitled to. In healthcare the issue is one of distributive justice – in other words, it is concerned with the distribution of goods, such as prescribing services in society. Beauchamp and Childress define justice as 'fair, equitable, and appropriate treatment in light of what is due or owed to persons' (Beauchamp & Childress 2013, p. 250).

This principle is highly relevant in debates about access to healthcare, prioritisation of patient care, rationing and providing care to individuals who are deemed to have contributed to their own health problems.

The principles in practice

Ethical principles can be very helpful when considering the issues that arise from ethical dilemmas. Suppose that Jane, a pharmacist prescriber with a conscientious objection to emergency hormonal contraception (EHC), refuses to prescribe the medication. Jane is professionally able to exercise her right to free determination and refuse to prescribe the medication, although the General Pharmaceutical Council does expect practitioners to refer patients to other providers in such circumstances (GPhC 2017b).

Jane can justify her actions morally by arguing that she is acting according to the principle of autonomy. However, the woman may argue that the pharmacist prescriber should respect her autonomous decision to have the EHC and prescribe it. But what other principles need to be considered here, as well as appealing to autonomy? Because Jane is refusing to prescribe the medication, the woman could be said to be seriously disadvantaged, and even harmed. Furthermore, the woman may argue that, in accordance with the principle of beneficence, the pharmacist is obliged to act for her benefit and avoid harm. Jane, on the other hand, may argue that she should not be obliged to provide a medication she has a conscientious objection to, because she considers the action of the medication to be harmful.

The key issue here is that neither the prescriber nor the woman agree on which act is harmful and which is beneficial. Competency 8 ('Prescribes professionally') includes statement 8.4: 'makes prescribing decisions based on the needs of patients and not the prescriber's personal considerations' (RPS 2016; see Appendix). How does this fit with Jane's decision? In Competency 10 ('Prescribe as part of a team'), it could be argued that there are others Jane can refer the patient to, but is this acceptable?

At first sight it may seem that an impasse has been reached but consider the position of one of the GPs in the practice or Jane's clinical line manager in a hospital where a moral decision had to be made to resolve the dilemma. How would taking account of the ethical principles help? The GP or line manager would need to decide who had the stronger claim to appeal to the principle of autonomy, and which act was considered to be beneficial and which harmful. This would enable actions to be justified with reference to the principles.

It might be decided, for example, that Jane was correct and was acting in accordance with the principle of autonomy, recognising that while the woman was entitled to receive EHC, her claim was not strong enough to override Jane's decision. Which act was considered to be harmful, and which beneficial, would also need to be taken into consideration. If it was thought that Jane was correct, acting according to the principles of beneficence and non-maleficence, it might be decided that while the woman would be inconvenienced, this degree of 'harm' was less than the 'harm' imposed on Jane should she be forced to prescribe medication she believed to be morally wrong.

What is important to note here is that it is unlikely a solution that is acceptable to both Jane and the woman can be found. This is a moral dilemma where all the possible solutions, by definition, are undesirable to at least one party affected by the decision. But referring to the ethical principles will give some structure to the discussion and will allow consideration of the pros and cons of each course of action. More importantly, it will give substantive reasons to justify and support the decisions taken, for which the prescriber may be held to account.

Summary of ethical considerations

Moral dilemmas are a recurring feature in clinical practice and pharmacist prescribers need to have the knowledge and skills required to solve the dilemmas they encounter. While inherent belief in what is right or wrong is important, practitioners will also need to be able to justify their chosen course of action if they are called to account by service users, their employers or regulatory body. Documents such as *In practice: Guidance on religion, personal values and beliefs* (GPhC 2017a) are important, but they do not give guidance for action in specific situations. The practitioner therefore needs to draw on other resources, such as the ethical theories outlined here. This section has focused on ethical principles in order to illustrate the application of theory to practice. However, other approaches and ways of thinking about these issues can be found in any standard text on healthcare or medical ethics and these are also worthy of consideration. While no theory can provide definitive instructions for action, it is incumbent on practitioners (as when they make clinical decisions) to reflect on ethical issues in a structured and formal way in order to reach a reasoned and justifiable decision.

Public health issues around prescribing

Competency 2 ('Consider the options') has statement 2.8, 'takes into account the wider perspective including the public health issues related to medicines and their use and promoting health'; and statement 2.19 'considers antimicrobial resistance and roles of infection control and stewardship'. According to the Faculty of Public Health, public health is 'The science and art of preventing disease, prolonging life and promoting health through organised efforts of society' (Acheson 1988). Public health practice is focused on improving the health of the population, rather than necessarily treating individual patients.

However public health is a collective duty of all health professionals. The business of attending to anticipatory care (helping people with long-term conditions plan their care) and discussing health promotion should be included whenever possible in every patient consultation or interaction. Anticipatory care can help reduce avoidable unscheduled acute admissions for people with pre-existing conditions, particularly older people, and those with mental health conditions.

Individual practitioners generally make a significant contribution to improving public health by advising on a range of important lifestyle areas that have significant health detriments such as smoking and alcohol. They also promote positive lifestyle choices such as regular exercise, healthy eating, and the safe use of medicines. Prescribers need a strategy to ensure that these discussions occur as part of every consultation and management plan, as described in Chapter 2.

Decisions made should benefit the individual without having a cost to society generally, as in the case of antimicrobial prescribing. Prescribing an antibiotic for one patient may reduce the efficacy of that antibiotic (through the process of resistance) for use in another patient. The individual needs of every patient should therefore be measured against the greater need to maintain the availability of antimicrobial agents for all, including future generations (O'Brien 2010). Use a local antibacterial formulary if possible or guidance from medicines management in the community or hospital to ensure that, from a public health perspective, prescribing is carried out within local antimicrobial guidelines.

Interestingly, some of these issues for non-medical prescribers were recognised over 10 years ago. In 2004, O'Brien argued that there was general acceptance that prescribers had an important role in 'managing public expectations of antimicrobial prescribing' and the result might therefore be a reduction in the amount of unnecessary prescriptions for antibiotics (O'Brien 2004). It is now recognised that a systematic process of judging (ignoring patient expectation) about whether or not to prescribe is likely to improve public health by preventing the prescribing of unnecessary antibiotics.

Likewise, Walsh (2006, S15) wrote:

> Giving public health advice and support may be of greater value than prescribing. The patient may not require a prescription but may benefit from purchasing an over-the-counter product. Prescription costs may be prohibitive for some patients and giving them a less expensive option should always be considered.

Competency 3 ('Reach a shared decision') includes statement 3.5, 'builds a relationship which encourages appropriate prescribing and not the expectation that a prescription will be supplied' (RPS 2016; see Appendix)

Alternative medicines, homeopathy, etc.

It is important to be aware that patients may have bought, or received, a wide range of 'alternative' medicines. There are many reasons why patients consider taking, for example, homeopathic preparations and, as with all aspects of prescribing, practitioners should listen and be sympathetic whatever their personal feelings and views may be. If patients have had poor experiences with conventional medicines they have received in the past, or their condition is not improving, they may turn to other forms of self-treatment.

As pharmacists using evidence-based medicine, it is very easy to argue against practices such as homeopathy but firstly it is important not to forget the power of the placebo effect; and secondly practitioners should always listen to the patient. However, there are some areas where alternative treatments are not only potentially dangerous for the individual but also the public at large. Examples of this would be homeopathic malaria prophylaxis or refusal of children's vaccinations. Individual pharmacists must ensure they use evidence-based medicine, are patient centred with a clear understanding of public health and patient care issues and be fully aware of the GPhC (2017b) Standards for pharmacy professionals.

Summary

This chapter has explored issues relating to the patient–prescriber partnership, including medication optimisation principles (encompassing appropriate and safe use of medications), the moral and ethical dilemmas facing patients and prescribers, and public health issues (including managing the use of alternative remedies). With all these issues, a common theme is the importance of effective communication during the consultation and the need for the prescriber to engage with the patient to elicit their preferences about how to manage their presenting complaint. Effectively engaging with the patient on these issues will enhance their involvement in the prescribing process, resulting in a collaborative management strategy on which patient and prescriber can agree and work together.

References

Acheson, Sir Donald, *et al.* (1988). *Public Health in England: The Report of the Committee of Inquiry into the Future Development of the Public Health Function.* London: HM Stationery Office.

Barber, N., Parsons, J. *et al.* (2004). Patients' problems with new medication for chronic conditions. *Quality and Safety in Health Care.* **13**(3), 172–75.

Beauchamp, T.L. & Childress, J.F. (2013). *Principles of Biomedical Ethics.* 7th edn. New York: Oxford University Press.

Bennett, C. (2010). *What is This Thing Called Ethics?* Oxford: Routledge.

Benson, A., Cribb, A. & Barber, N. (2009). Understanding pharmacists' values: A qualitative study of ideals and dilemmas in UK pharmacy practice. *Social Science and Medicine.* **68**(12), 2223–30.

Carter, Lord (2016). *Operational productivity and performance in English NHS acute hospitals: Unwarranted variations.* https://assets.publishing.service.gov.uk/government/uploads/system/uploads/attachment_data/file/499229/Operational_productivity_A.pdf (last accessed 20.5.2019).

Chew, K. (2013). *Animals Helped Make Your Medicine: What Can a Vegan Do?* https://www.care2.com/causes/animals-helped-make-your-medicine-what-can-a-vegan-do-2.html (last accessed 20.5.2019).

Datapharm (2019). *Electronic Medicine Compendium.* https://www.medicines.org.uk/emc (last accessed 16.5.2019).

Department of Health (DH) (2015). *The NHS Constitution.* London: Department of Health.

Doyle, C., Lennox, L. & Bell, D. (2013). A systematic review of evidence on the links between patient experience and clinical safety and effectiveness. *British Medical Journal Open.* **3**(1), e001570.

Duerden, M., Avery, A. & Payne, R. (2013). *Polypharmacy and Medicines Optimisation: Making it Safe and Sound.* The King's Fund. https://www.kingsfund.org.uk/sites/default/files/field/field_publication_file/polypharmacy-and-medicines-optimisation-kingsfund-nov13.pdf (last accessed 20.5.2019).

Fortin, M., Bravo, G., *et al.* (2005). Prevalence of multi-morbidity among adults seen in family practice. *Annals of Family Medicine.* **3**(3), 223–28.

General Pharmaceutical Council (GPhC) (2016). *Prescribers Survey Report.* https://www.pharmacyregulation.org/sites/default/files/gphc_prescribers_survey_report.pdf (last accessed 14.5.2019).

General Pharmaceutical Council (GPhC) (2017a). *Standards for pharmacy professionals.* London: GPhC.

General Pharmaceutical Council (GPhC) (2017b). *In practice: Guidance on religion, personal values and beliefs.* https://www.pharmacyregulation.org/sites/default/files/in_practice-_guidance_on_religion_personal_values_and_beliefs.pdf (last accessed 28.5.2019).

Gillon, R. (1985). Conscience, good character, integrity, and to hell with philosophical medical ethics? *British Medical Journal.* **290**(6480), 1497–98.

Harris, J. (1985). *The Value of Life.* London: Routledge.

Horne. R., Chapman. S., *et al.* (2013) Understanding patients' adherence-related beliefs about medicines prescribed for long-term conditions: a meta-analytic review of the Necessity-Concerns Framework. *PLoS One.* **8**(12), e80633.

Mair, F. (2014). Thinking about the burden of treatment. *British Medical Journal.* **349**, g6680.

Mason, J. (2013). Medicines optimisation – it's everybody's business. *Prescriber.* **24**(7), 40–42.

Medicines and Healthcare products Regulatory Agency (MHRA) (2019). *Yellow Card Scheme.* https://yellowcard.mhra.gov.uk/ (last accessed 20.5.2019).

NRLS (2019). National Reporting and Learning System. NHS Improvement. https://improvement.nhs.uk/resources/learning-from-patient-safety-incidents/ (last accessed 20.5.2019).

National Institute for Health and Care Excellence (NICE) (2015). *Medicines optimisation: the safe and effective use of medicines to enable the best possible outcomes.* https://www.sps.nhs.uk/wp-content/uploads/2015/06/Presn_from_MUSN_Mtg_25_June_15_MO20guidelines_LP.pdf (last accessed 20.5.2019).

National Institute for Health and Care Excellence (NICE) (2016). *Medicines Optimisation – Quality Standard 120.* https://www.nice.org.uk/guidance/qs120/resources/medicines-optimisation-pdf-75545351857861 (last accessed 20.5.2019).

O'Brien, S.J. (2004). 'Extended/supplementary prescribing: a public health perspective. Antimicrobial Resistance'. In: M. Courtenay & M. Griffiths (eds). *Independent and Supplementary Prescribing: An Essential Guide.* London: Greenwich Medical Media.

O'Brien, S.J. (2010). 'Extended/supplementary prescribing: a public health perspective'. In: M. Courtenay & M. Griffiths (eds). *Independent and Supplementary Prescribing: An Essential Guide*. Cambridge: Cambridge University Press.

Pirmohamed, M., James, S., Meakin, S. *et al.* (2004). Adverse drug reactions as cause of admission to hospital: prospective analysis of 18 820 patients. *British Medical Journal*. **329**, 15.

Queensland Department of Health (DOH) (2013) *Department of Health Guideline for the Use of Medicines/Pharmaceuticals of Animal Origin*. Queensland, Australia. https://www.health.qld.gov.au/__data/assets/pdf_file/0024/147507/qh-gdl-954.pdf (last accessed 20.5.2019).

Royal College of General Practitioners (RCGP) (2013). *Managing multi-morbidity in practice... what lessons can be learnt from the care of people with COPD and co-morbidities?* https://www.educationforhealth.org/wp-content/uploads/2015/03/COPD_MultiMorbidities.pdf (last accessed 20.5.2019).

Royal Pharmaceutical Society (RPS) (2013). Medicines Optimisation: Helping patients to make the most of medicines. Good practice guidance for healthcare professionals in England. https://www.rpharms.com/Portals/0/RPS%20 document%20library/Open%20access/Policy/helping-patients-make-the-most-of-their-medicines.pdf (last accessed 20.5.2019).

Royal Pharmaceutical Society (RPS) (2016). *A Competency Framework for All Prescribers*. London: RPS. https://www.rpharms.com/Portals/0/RPS%20document%20library/Open%20access/Professional%20standards/Prescribing%20 competency%20framework/prescribing-competency-framework.pdf (last accessed 14.5.2019).

Trueman, P., Lowson, K., Blighe, A., *et al.* (2010). *Evaluation of the Scale, Causes and Costs of Waste Medicines: Final Report*. York: University of York.

Walsh, J. (2006). Non-medical prescribing in nurse-led community leg ulcer clinics. *British Journal of Nursing*. **15** (11), S14–16.

World Health Organisation (WHO) (1995). The Judicially Prohibited and Impure Substances in Foodstuffs and Drugs. http://www.immunize.org/talking-about-vaccines/porcine.pdf (last accessed 20.5.2019).

5

Prescribing for specific groups of patients

Afthab Hussain

Chapter overview

This chapter will cover prescribing for patients within 'specialist' groups, including:

- Neonates and children
- Older people
- Pregnant women
- Breast-feeding women
- Patients with chronic renal impairment
- Patients with chronic hepatic impairment.

The aim of the chapter is to explain the factors that change within these 'specialist' patient groups and help the prescriber to prescribe safely for them. It will also provide an insight into the principles that should be followed and highlight reliable sources of information that should be consulted when deciding to prescribe medicines for these patient groups, and considering whether and how doses need to be adjusted.

Introduction

In the *Competency Framework for All Prescribers*, Competency 2, 'Consider the options' (RPS 2016; see Appendix), a number of issues are highlighted. These include, for example, assessing how comorbidities can impact on the management options, as in statement 2.4: 'applies understanding of the mode of action and pharmacokinetics of medicines and how these may be altered by e.g. genetics, age, renal impairment and pregnancy'. Also, in Competency 1 ('Assess the patient'), the concepts discussed below make the requirements of the Competency relevant.

Pharmacists are aware that within these 'specialist' patient groups there are potential changes in pharmacokinetics and pharmacodynamics and therefore particular care and attention is required before prescribing for any of them. Patients within these groups are more likely to experience adverse drug reactions and are associated with higher than average prescribing errors.

Prescribing for neonates and children

Children (or, more specifically, neonates) differ in their response to drugs, compared to adults. There is a limited amount of research available in children and neonates to determine the effectiveness of medicines in healthy and ill children. It is important, therefore, not to generalise information from adult studies to paediatric populations, as this may lead to serious errors. When prescribing for neonates (in the first 28 days after birth), for example, extra care should be taken to calculate the correct dose.

There are also significant differences in drug pharmacokinetics between paediatric patients and adults. Selecting the correct dose is critical, due to the wide variation in weight and physical development from birth through to the age of 18. These physiological changes affect drug absorption, distribution, metabolism and excretion.

Pharmacokinetic changes occurring in paediatric patients

Absorption

As a child grows and develops, their absorption of drugs generally becomes more efficient. Neonates have less developed absorption and prescribers need to take this into account. Overall, the bioavailability of a drug (the amount reaching the systemic circulation) is the same but the onset of action of the drug may be delayed, due to the rate of absorption being reduced in very young children.

Generally, gastric emptying is slower in young children compared to adults and this is the case for the first six months of life. Other factors that can affect drug absorption include hydration status, poor nutritional habits and underlying gastrointestinal disease.

The absorption of topical creams and emollients in children may be significantly increased, as the stratum corneum (outermost layer of the skin) is much thinner and more porous. The body surface area to weight ratio is much higher in neonates and consequently leads to a greater risk of adverse effects.

Another consideration is muscle mass. Neonates lack muscle mass and the use of intramuscular (IM) injections should therefore be avoided as it can be very painful. Also, the absorption of drugs from an IM injection can be unpredictable, as there is variability in systemic blood flow. In addition, conditions and illnesses that lead to hypermotility in the gastrointestinal tract, and that may also be associated with vomiting or diarrhoea, may reduce drug absorption.

Distribution

A number of factors can affect drug distribution. These might include body fluid, tissue composition and protein-binding capability. In neonates, body composition is about 70% water and, as the child grows, this is reduced to between 50 and 60%. From childbirth to 1 year, body fat content rises from 12 to 30%. Administration of water-soluble drugs, like gentamycin, require larger doses (mg/kg) in neonates, compared to older children, to ensure that therapeutic levels are reached systemically.

As a drug is absorbed, some of it is bound to plasma proteins circulating throughout the body – mainly albumin and glycoproteins. Some of the drug remains unbound and free. This unbound, free drug is able to cross cell membranes and bind to its target to induce a response. Neonates and children have lower levels of plasma proteins (such as albumin) than adults; they also have lower levels of protein binding sites. This means that more of the drug is available to exert its physiological effect and thus leads to lower doses being required.

Metabolism

Drug metabolism is mainly carried out by the liver, with some metabolism occurring in the kidneys and lungs. The liver is not fully developed until the age of 6–13 months. Drug metabolism, in general, is therefore reduced in neonates and very young children. As the child grows, metabolic activity is increased. Children between 1 and 5 years of age may therefore require larger doses, or less time between doses of the drug.

Excretion

Drug excretion occurs in the lungs, sweat glands and salivary glands but mainly in the kidneys. Renal function in neonates is significantly less than in a child or adult. After the age of 1, renal function is much better than adults and over time it slowly declines. As a result of decreased renal function, drugs are eliminated slowly from the body and can accumulate and cause toxicity.

Sources of information about dosing

To determine the correct dose of a drug for neonates and children, consult the *Paediatric and Neonatal Dosage Handbook* (Taketomo, Hodding, Kraus 2017–18). The British National Formulary (Pharmaceutical Press 2019) indicates doses for adults and some doses for children. To prescribe in children, the gold standard source of information is the BNF for Children (BNF-C) (Paediatric Formulary Committee 2017–2018).

Calculating doses in paediatrics

In the *Competency Framework,* Competency 4 ('Prescribe'), includes statement 4.6: 'accurately completes and routinely checks calculations relevant to prescribing and practical dosing' (RPS 2016; see Appendix). To calculate the dose of a drug in paediatric patients, there are three main methods: body weight, body surface area and dosing by age.

Body weight

In paediatrics, dosing based on a child's body weight is the most common method used to calculate doses. In the BNF-C doses are shown as mg/kg body weight (Paediatric Formulary Committee 2017–2018). A prescription for a paediatric patient should always include the body weight of the patient to allow pharmacy staff to double-check and reduce the potential for errors. As a guide, the dose in paediatric patients should never exceed that of an adult patient. For example, if the dose of a given drug is 10mg/kg (maximum dose 350mg), a child weighing 10kg should receive a dose of 100mg, but a child weighing 40kg should receive a dose of 350mg (rather than 400mg). There has been an increase in obesity in children so, when dealing with these patients prescribers should consider using the mean weight for a child that age (see the section at the back of the BNF-C to determine mean height and weight for a child). The short BNF-C section is entitled 'Prescribing for children: weight, height and gender' and this is covered in Competency 2 ('Consider the options'), statement 2.4: 'applies understanding of the mode of action and pharmacokinetics of medicines and how these may be altered (e.g. by genetics, age, renal impairment, pregnancy)' (RPS 2016; see Appendix).

Doses required to treat a particular illness are often expressed as a single dose accompanied by a frequency of doses (e.g. 2mg/kg three times a day). In some cases, doses are stated as a total daily dose, e.g. 10mg/kg in two divided doses. Prescribers should therefore take extra care to determine whether the recommendations are stated as total daily doses or single doses to avoid the risk of overdose.

Body surface area

Body surface area (BSA) can also be used with physiological parameters to determine drug handling. BSA can be calculated using nomograms with the child's weight (under or over 40kg) although this can be difficult to calculate in severely ill children. It is used when prescribing a limited number of drugs – for example, cytotoxic anti-cancer drugs. At the back of the BNF-C there is a table that allows practitioners to determine BSA according to body weight. This table is entitled 'Body Surface Area in Children' and it goes from a 1kg child to a 90kg child.

Age

Many drugs have a wide therapeutic range and are quoted as a single dose for a particular age group. For example, for paracetamol, the neonate oral dose at 28–32 weeks corrected gestational age is 20 mg/kg as a single dose, then 10–15 mg/kg every 8–12 hours as required, with a maximum dose of 30 mg/kg daily in divided doses. Similarly, in a child aged 1–2 months the dose is 30–60mg every 8 hours as required, with a maximum dose of 60 mg/kg per day in divided doses. Children who are underweight for their age need a dose adjustment to avoid the risk of overdose. Practitioners should therefore use the 'mean values for weight by age tables', which can be found at the back of the BNF-C, as a guide.

Although all three methods can be used, prescribers must ensure that the dose calculated can be practically measured. Standard liquid medicines prescribed at under 5ml doses are accompanied with 5ml oral syringes that have 0.5ml divisions highlighted. Prescribing 3.25ml of a drug would therefore be difficult to correctly administer. Other sizes of oral syringes may also be available. For example, a 5ml spoon is supplied for doses of 5ml or multiples of 5ml.

Other factors to consider when prescribing for children

Excipients

Wherever possible, sugar-free preparations should be prescribed and these are listed in the BNF-C under each monograph as appropriate. Some liquid preparations contain high levels of alcohol and are therefore unsuitable for children. For instance, benzyl alcohol (a preservative) is sometimes found in injectable products and should be avoided in neonates, as its administration has been shown to be associated with foetal syndrome (also known as gasping syndrome in pre-term neonates). There is a section entitled 'Excipients', at the beginning of the BNF-C in the 'Guidance on prescribing', which covers these.

Using unlicensed medicines

Many prescribed paediatric preparations are used outside their licence (or off-label), and only licensed for use in adults. This is because manufacturers will only investigate the drugs' efficacy and safety in adults during clinical trials – often due to difficulty in recruiting children. In general, up to three-quarters of prescribed medicines on paediatric wards are used clinically outside their licence (Shah *et al.* 2007). Care should be taken when prescribing medicines outside their licence, as this increases individual professional responsibility and liability. Prescribers can find reliable information in paediatric units, which will often have clear, reliable reference materials provided by the manufacturers themselves.

Medication adherence in children

There are a number of factors that can contribute to poor adherence to prescribed medication in children, including lack of parental support, unattractive preparation, poor taste, poor instructions, and parental concerns regarding efficacy and side effects. These factors should be discussed with the parents and reasonable adjustments made by the prescriber to improve adherence, such as suggesting a specific flavour or an alternative administration route (Laforgia *et al.* 2014).

Prescribing in older people

Older people have higher rates of chronic illness and are therefore more likely to be taking multiple medicines, which is referred to as polypharmacy (Bokhof & Junius-Walker 2016). Polypharmacy is also discussed in Chapter 4. With better healthcare systems, including improved and early diagnosis and treatment, the number of over-65s has increased by 47% since 1974, currently accounting for 18% of the total population within the UK. Furthermore, there has been an 89% increase in the number of over-75s, who currently account for over 8% of the UK population (Office for National Statistics 2018).

Competency 4, in the *Competency Framework*, is entitled 'Prescribe' and includes statement 4.2: 'understands the potential for adverse effects and takes steps to avoid/minimise, recognise and manage them' (RPS 2016; see Appendix). In general, elderly patients have a higher incidence of comorbidities, with an associated higher use of medication. At the same time, as we age, there are significant changes in pharmacokinetics and pharmacodynamics. Taken together, these factors potentially increase the risk of adverse drug reactions and interactions. Care must therefore be taken when prescribing for this potentially vulnerable group.

Pharmacokinetic changes in the aging patient

Distribution

The proportion of body fat increases and water content decreases during the aging process. With increased body fat content in elderly patients, fat-soluble drugs are distributed into a larger pool, subsequently prolonging the half-life of the drug and increasing the time taken to clear the drug from the body. This increases the risk of drug accumulation if the dose is not adjusted. For instance, benzodiazepine nitrazepam has a half-life of 30 hours in adults but this increases to 40 hours in elderly patients. Prescribing this medication for older patients would therefore lead to prolonged effects of sedation the next morning, increasing the risks of confusion and falls (Obayashi *et al.* 2013).

With decreased water content, administering the same dose as adults will result in increased serum levels in older people. Examples of drugs where increased serum levels are seen include digoxin and gentamycin.

Excretion

The kidney is the main organ responsible for drug excretion. Renal function is known to decline during the aging process, at a rate of about 1% per year, although there is wide variation between patients (Viazzi *et al.* 2016). More recently, comorbidities (including hypertension and diabetes) have been shown to impact negatively on renal function. It is therefore imperative to monitor renal function in older people and adjust doses accordingly. The requirement to consider and review the potential impact of excretion changes on prescribing decisions is covered in Competency 1 ('Assess the patient').

Existing chronic renal failure or diabetes can lead to a decline in renal function when using non-steroidal anti-inflammatory drugs (NSAIDs), including ibuprofen. As mentioned in Chapter 2, when taking a patient history the practitioner needs to determine the use of over-the-counter medications, such as NSAIDs, alongside prescribed medication.

Metabolism

The prevalence of chronic liver disease is increasing in the elderly population (Michielson & Vandewoude 2010). During the aging process, there is a decrease in liver volume and hepatic blood flow. The liver has a large reserve volume so (despite the physiological changes that occur with aging) there is usually no need to adjust the dose of hepatically metabolised drugs – unless there is underlying liver disease.

Pharmacodynamic changes in the aging patient

Compared to younger adults, older people are known to be more sensitive to drugs (Bowie & Slattum. 2007). Elderly patients are also more vulnerable to the adverse effects of their medicines, due to reduced drug elimination, impaired renal function, increased sensitivity of organs to drugs, and multi-drug interactions in polypharmacy.

Elderly patients are also less likely to receive the maximum benefit of drugs, due to potential poor adherence to medication regimens, forgetfulness associated with cognitive decline and difficulty swallowing (see also Chapter 4). Some of the common adverse effects are described below. These all link to Competency 2 ('Consider options'), particularly statement 2.4 'understanding how pharmacokinetics might change', statement 2.5 which considers comorbidities, and statement 2.6: 'takes into account any relevant patient factors (e.g. ability to swallow)' (RPS 2016; see Appendix).

Postural hypotension and imbalance

Elderly patients are known to exhibit signs of postural hypotension due to age-related impaired homeostatic responses (Figueroa *et al.* 2010). Drugs that affect the cardiovascular system are more likely to result in postural hypotension and subsequently to an increase in the risk of falls (Torstensson *et al.* 2015). Central nervous system depressants, such as benzodiazepines and opiates, are also known to decrease sympathetic flow and raise the risk of falls. The increased risk of falls in elderly patients is also associated with increased morbidity and mortality. Medication reviews are therefore critical, when treating elderly patients, to reduce these risks (Stubbs *et al.* 2015). Drugs like benzodiazepines, opiates and some antidepressants can also lead to balance problems in elderly patients and can further contribute to the risk of falls.

Cognitive function

Medicines that act on the central nervous system can negatively affect cognitive abilities. Opiates, some antidepressants, antipsychotics and benzodiazepines are all known to impair cognitive function in elderly patients. The cholinergic system plays a central role in cognitive function so drugs that exert anticholinergic effects (such as amitriptyline, oxybutynin and hyoscine) may lead to confusion and exacerbate cognitive dysfunction in those with pre-existing cognitive decline. Patients presenting with acute confusion or delirium should always undergo a medication review to determine whether their medication is the cause. To this end, Competency 1 ('Assess the patient') includes elements of medication and clinical history taking as well as clinical assessment prior to prescribing (RPS 2016; see Appendix).

Visceral muscle function

Constipation is common in elderly patients and can often be attributed to drug therapy. A number of medicines can cause constipation, including opiates, anticholinergics and tricyclic antidepressants. Medications should be reviewed to determine whether they are the cause before adding medication to treat constipation. This again emphasises the importance of the medication review (see Chapter 2).

Conditions such as benign prostatic hypertrophy (which is common in elderly males) can also cause urinary retention and this may be exacerbated by using inhaled anticholinergic drugs like ipratropium bromide or tiotropium bromide, which are prescribed to reduce smooth muscle contraction in the respiratory system (Loke & Singh 2010).

Elderly people may also have bladder problems such as urge or stress incontinence. These symptoms are exacerbated in patients who are prescribed diuretics, which increase the incidence of urinary incontinence. It is important to inform the patient of the effects of such medication and discuss the best time to take their dose, as a late evening dose will lead to diuresis through the night which will affect sleep. Competency 3 ('Reach a shared decision') may lead to the patient deciding the offered treatment is not appropriate for them at this time and other options may need to be considered (RPS 2016; see Appendix).

Other high-risk medications in the elderly

A number of other important medications need to be used with caution in elderly people.

Warfarin

Anticoagulants such as warfarin, though often essential, need to be used with care in older people, who often require lowering doses. The standard loading dose of warfarin in younger adults, for example, is 10mg but in older people this is reduced to 5mg. To ensure that warfarin is used safely, regular International Normalised Ratio tests (INRs) are required to adjust future doses. In patients with cognitive impairment or confusion, it may be difficult to retrieve appropriate blood samples or ensure regimen adherence. It is therefore critical to ensure that appropriate support is in place to ensure safe use of such medication.

Non-steroidal anti-inflammatory drugs (NSAIDs)

Older people are at higher risk of gastrointestinal bleeding (GI) where the risk is further increased with the use of non-steroidal anti-inflammatories (NSAIDs) (Pilotto & Franceschi 2003). In 2000, Kaplan noted that 1% of those aged over 80 years of age are hospitalised with GI bleeding (Kaplan *et al.* 2001), though this may have improved with the increased use of proton pump inhibitors (PPIs). NSAIDs have also been shown to reduce renal function, exacerbate heart failure and increase the risk of a heart attack or stroke.

A number of studies have shown that PPIs such as omeprazole and lansoprazole should be prescribed alongside NSAIDs to reduce the risk of GI bleeding (Scheiman 2013). For prescribers, it is particularly important to review the use of NSAIDs in elderly people. Are NSAIDs clinically necessary for this particular patient? Long-term use makes the patient most vulnerable and prescribers must attempt to minimise the risks while maintaining patient confidence and attempting to reduce the pain and inflammation.

Hypoglycaemic drugs

The prevalence of Type 2 diabetes increases as we age and this condition is commonly treated with oral hypoglycaemic drugs. Not surprisingly, one of the most serious adverse effects of these drugs is hypoglycaemia which, if left untreated, leads to increased morbidity and mortality. Glibenclamide, a long-acting sulfonylurea, causes an increase in blood insulin levels and can lead to hypoglycaemia. In older people, short-acting hypoglycaemic drugs such as gliclazide should be considered first, to reduce these risks.

Hypoglycaemia is under-reported in older people and the incidence of such episodes should be documented. When prescribing or modifying the dose of hypoglycaemic drugs, care should be taken to ensure that the patient is informed of the risks of hypoglycaemia and how it should be treated and managed. Competency 5, 'Provide information' (RPS 2016; see Appendix), stresses the need to provide information but also to check that the patient understands what to do if side effects develop – particularly hypoglycaemia. Patients should be advised of the signs and symptoms of hypoglycaemia. Where hypoglycaemia is suspected, blood sugars should be checked. If possible, patients should be given 15–20g carbohydrates (NICE 2017) to counteract the effect.

Other risk factors in elderly patients

Polypharmacy

As older people are more likely to have multiple illnesses, the number of medications they take also potentially increases. Regular reviews of the appropriateness of medication are critical.

Furthermore, in older people with intellectual disability and/or cognitive decline, the risks from polypharmacy are more prevalent (Messerli *et al.* 2016). It is also important to document the use of over-the-counter medications to identify potential risks and drug interactions with prescribed medications and food (Ewen *et al.* 2015). See also Chapter 2 which looks at information gathering during the consultation.

Hospital discharge

Following hospital admission, a number of changes may be made to a patient's medicine prescription, including the addition or removal of drugs, or perhaps a change in dose frequency. Competency 4 ('Prescribe'), includes statement 4.13 'communicates information about medicines and what they are being used for when sharing or transferring prescribing responsibilities/ information' and statement 10.1 'acts as part of a team to ensure continuity of care across care settings' (RPS 2016; see Appendix). These competencies are of particular importance when the patient is discharged so that information reaches the primary care practitioner prior to the patient's next visit.

Physical factors

Hearing and vision decline in older people and this may affect the patient's ability to listen, read and understand information relating to taking their medication correctly. Information leaflets, found with prescribed medicines, are often in a small font that visually impaired people have difficulty in reading. In such cases, patients should be provided with leaflets in large print wherever possible. Prescribers can obtain these for patients by ringing the Royal National Institute of Blind People (RNIB) Medicine Leaflet Line on 0800 198 5000. The prescriber will need the name of the medicine and the medicine's product license or marketing authorisation number (normally a 9-figure number prefaced with the letters PL, MA or EU, which can be found on the medicine packaging). Always check the patient's understanding of, and commitment to, the medicines that are being suggested and arrange management, monitoring and follow-up in line with Competency 5, 'Provide information' (RPS 2016; see Appendix).

Older people often also have weaker manual dexterity, which can affect their ability to take their medication – for example, they may have difficulty opening blister packs or removing lids from bottles. Inhalers may cause problems for the same reason. The older patient's needs should be considered, and an appropriate alternative provided where possible. Some elderly people have difficulty swallowing tablets due to dysphagia and they should be provided with liquid preparations where possible and practical. Involve the local community pharmacy, as they can usually offer support.

Cognitive function

In patients with impaired cognitive function (for example, due to stroke, dementia or Alzheimer's disease), adhering to a medication plan may be problematic. It is important that medication plans are discussed with carers to ensure adherence. It is also important to note that disorientation, confusion or depression can add to risk factors for medicines-related problems and should always be considered as a potential cause of impaired cognitive function.

Social support

Many older patients may have carers who help care for them and assist them with taking their medications. Throughout the Competency Framework, carers are included alongside patients in the competencies. Where such care is in place, it is important to inform the carers of any changes to the medication plan. Competency 5 includes statement 5.4 'ensures that the patient/carer knows what to do if there are any concerns about the management of their condition if the condition deteriorates or if there is no improvement in a specific time frame' and Competency 3, 'Reach a shared decision' (RPS 2016; see Appendix), covers the same issues. In older people who are independent, there is an increased risk of problems arising. In such cases, where it is thought the patient may be at risk, it is important for the multidisciplinary team to discuss how to put in place the best support and plan of action to reduce the risk for the patient.

Prescribing in pregnancy

Prescribing for pregnant women should be avoided where possible, as drugs can affect a foetus at any stage of its development including after the baby is born. Pregnant women may require treatment for pre-existing conditions such as asthma, epilepsy, diabetes, hypertension and hypothyroidism. Pregnant women may also require treatment for conditions that arise as a result of the pregnancy, such as gestational diabetes, hypertension and morning sickness.

Competency 7 ('Prescribe safely') includes statement 7.1: 'prescribes within own scope of practice and recognises the limits of own knowledge and skill'. If prescribing for a pregnant patient, this is particularly important. It is necessary to consider the benefits and risks of prescribing for both the mother and the foetus. There are also risks associated with prescribing for women of child-bearing age – for example, if the patient is taking anti-epilepsy medication, there is a risk of the medication causing structural, behavioural and functional changes to the foetus should the patient become pregnant.

As is mentioned again in Chapter 6, female patients with epilepsy who are of child-bearing age must no longer be prescribed valproate unless they have a pregnancy prevention programme in place (MHRA 2018). Other anti-epileptics, such as carbamazepine and lamotrigine, are known to increase the risk of the foetus developing malformations including cleft palate (Pennell 2016) Prescribers must make sure that such female patients with epilepsy seek further advice before conceiving. Medicines Information Services are shown on the inside cover of the BNF. The local service will be able to contact specialist units that deal specifically with medicines queries for pregnant and breast-feeding women.

Many drugs are known to cause congenital malformations, including structural, behavioural and functional changes to the foetus, and these are described as teratogenic. It is difficult to assess the potential teratogenic effects of drugs, as pregnant women are excluded from clinical trials for ethical reasons. As a result, the teratogenic effects of drugs are retrieved from case reports or epidemiological studies. Around 1–2% of congenital malformations are associated with drugs and therefore no drug can be deemed safe in pregnancy. Established drugs are generally considered safer and prescribed preferentially, compared with newer agents. However, as mentioned above, some of the older drugs (for example, the ones used to treat epilepsy) are specifically banned for this group of patients.

If necessary, Medicines Information Services in the local hospital can be contacted, as they have access to specialist medicines information. If a particular medicine is unlicensed in pregnant women, some confidence can still be gained from the data kept by the Medicines Information Services. Another possible source of information is the Medicines Information Unit of the company that makes the medicine. They will have examples of it being used or they may advise a change in therapy to minimise risk. Pregnant women with epilepsy, for example, cannot be left without treatment but expert opinion is required to ensure the safety of mother and baby. The telephone numbers for manufacturers are in the BNF or on medicines.org.uk (Datapharm 2019).

Timing of prescribing

From conception to about the eighth week of gestation, drugs can lead to failure of implantation and miscarriage. It is important to note the exact day of conception, as – if there is uncertainty – extra vigilance is needed.

The embryonic phase (days 18–55) is considered the high-risk period, as damage occurring during this stage is associated with congenital malformations. During the foetal period (day 56 to birth), there is organ development and maturation and these processes can still be adversely affected by drugs. Damage occurring during this stage has been associated with functional damage, e.g. deafness.

Prescribing in the last trimester of pregnancy may result in pharmacological effects in the neonate. Consider the risks compared with the benefits or consider, where clinically acceptable, delaying the prescription until after the birth.

Drugs requiring extra caution during pregnancy:

- Beta-blockers – known to lead to low birth weights
- Sulfonylureas – can cause foetal hypoglycaemia
- Opioid analgesics – can cause neonatal respiratory depression
- Antidepressants – if taking paroxetine and planning pregnancy, stop taking the drug
- Anxiolytics – benzodiazepines should not be routinely prescribed
- Valproate and other drugs used in epilepsy
- Polypharmacy increases the risk of teratogenicity.

If pregnant patients are prescribed medicines that may (or definitely will) affect the neonate, the patient should be referred to a consultant for long-term care and follow-up. This will reduce the risk of adverse effects to the neonate. Competency 7 ('Prescribe safely') includes statement 7.1, which reminds all prescribers to prescribe within their own scope of practice and recognise the limits of their own knowledge and skills (RPS 2016; see Appendix).

Pharmacokinetic changes during pregnancy

During pregnancy, the blood volume can increase by up to 50%, thus increasing the drug distribution volume. Renal function is also known to increase by about 50%. Clearance of drugs that are excreted by the kidneys may therefore be affected. Drugs with narrow therapeutic indices, such as digoxin, phenytoin and carbamazepine, need to be monitored closely and will require regular monitoring (Meader & Loring 2016, Panchaud *et al.* 2014).

Drugs with teratogenic effects are discussed in Chapter 6.

The key principles for reducing risk in pregnancy are:

- Where possible avoid drug use in the first trimester or seek expert advice where this is not possible
- Assess the benefits and risks to both the mother and foetus if drugs are withheld
- Use well-established drugs with good safety profiles and avoid newer medications
- Avoid valproate and use other drugs to treat epilepsy with great caution and under expert supervision
- Avoid multi-drug use where possible
- Avoid known teratogenic drugs where possible or seek expert advice where this is not possible
- Discuss the adverse effects of drugs in women of child-bearing age and discuss the use of effective contraception
- Use the lowest effective dose where possible and for the shortest period possible
- For drugs with narrow therapeutic indices, consider regular monitoring and dose adjustment and consider referring to the consultant for long-term care.

Some drugs have effects later in pregnancy. For instance, tetracyclines taken during pregnancy stain the teeth of children; and this staining can be permanent. During childbirth, salbutamol, calcium channel blockers and NSAIDs have tocolytic (labour-suppressing) effects. Neonates may also experience respiratory depression due to opioid analgesics being used by the pregnant mother during pregnancy.

Sources of information for drugs in pregnancy

The BNF (Joint Formulary Committee) provides useful information regarding the use of medications in pregnancy. Much of this is under the monograph of each specific drug or at the beginning of the section where the drugs under consideration can be found. Further information can be obtained from the UK Teratology Information Service (UKTIS) or TOXBASE (www.toxbase.org) which provides expert advice and guidance on the adverse effects of drugs. As mentioned above, medicines information services and the drug companies themselves can be very helpful.

Prescribing for breast-feeding mothers

Breast-feeding mothers being prescribed medicines are often concerned about the effects, if any, the drugs will have on the neonate and on very young children. Therefore, it is important to understand and explain the benefits and risks to the mother. Ultimately, the aim is to protect the neonate and young child from adverse drug effects from maternal medication that may pass to the baby in the breast milk. Where possible, medicines should be used where the mother may continue breast-feeding without risk to the child. Breast-feeding should be encouraged where possible and research has shown that breast milk is the most beneficial feed for a neonate (Victora & Bahl 2016).

Maternal medication often passes into the breast milk, though the dose the neonate receives is often low and below any therapeutic level. The BNF is a useful guide, although manufacturers often say that the drug should be avoided in breast-feeding, when there is little information. The

Summary of Product Characteristics (SmPC) has a section on breast-feeding as it relates to each of its included medicines. These can be found at medicines.org.uk (Datapharm 2019).

General principles

There are a number of key principles that should be followed to reduce the risk of infants being exposed to potentially toxic drugs during breast-feeding:

- Avoid unnecessary maternal drug use
- Avoid the use of complementary or alternative medicines due to the limited availability of research and data on their effects
- Assess over-the-counter medication use
- Assess benefit versus risk on a patient by patient basis
- If the drug is appropriate for use, prescribe the lowest dose over the shortest term possible
- Consider local preparations (topical/inhaled) that result in lower maternal plasma concentrations and subsequent lower expression in maternal milk
- In drugs that have a short half-life, advise the patient to take the dose after feeding to reduce peak drug concentrations
- Avoid newer drugs unless there is clear information about their safety in breast-feeding
- Prescribe drugs with better safety profiles in breast-feeding mothers
- Ask patients to stop breast-feeding while taking cytotoxic agents or seek specialist advice
- Monitor the infant for adverse drug effects.

Sources of information on drugs in breast milk

The BNF (Pharmaceutical Press 2019) provides basic information on drug prescribing in pregnancy and in breast feeding. The Summary of Product Characteristics (SmPC) has a section on breast-feeding as it relates to each of its included medicines. These can be found at medicines.org.uk (Datapharm 2019) and will often advise caution. Local Medicines Information Services can generally be a good source of detailed information. The BNF offers advice but is by no means definitive.

Patients with renal impairment

A knowledge of pharmacokinetics and an ability to use the BNF will prepare prescribers for the patient with any form of renal impairment. The *Competency Framework*, particularly Competency 2 ('Consider the options'), and statement 2.4, expects all prescribers to 'apply an understanding of the mode of action and pharmacokinetics of medicines and to take account of genetics, age, renal impairment and pregnancy' (RPS 2016; see Appendix). Patients with impaired renal function are identified by calculating the estimated glomerular filtration rate (eGFR). Patients with a persistent eGFR of <60ml/min will be categorised as having impaired renal function.

As discussed previously, renal function is known to decline with age so a significant proportion of elderly patients will have some degree of renal impairment. Where there is underlying renal impairment and the drugs prescribed are renally eliminated, accumulation of the drug or its metabolites can occur, and subsequent doses may need reducing. The level of renal function below which the dose of a drug must be reduced depends on its toxicity and the proportion of the drug eliminated by renal excretion. For many drugs with only minor or no dose-related side-effects, very precise modification of the dose regimen is unnecessary and a simple scheme for dose reduction is sufficient. In treating patients with renal impairment, the daily maintenance dose of a drug can be reduced – either by reducing the size of the dose or by increasing the time between doses.

A number of commonly prescribed drugs require caution in patients with underlying renal impairment. These include metformin, ACE inhibitors, angiotensin receptor blockers, spironolactone, NSAIDs, atenolol, allopurinol, methotrexate and aminoglycosides. It may be possible to reduce doses or it may be necessary to change the treatment completely.

Estimation of renal function

The degree of renal impairment needs to be considered before the dose is adjusted. Two methods are commonly used to estimate the degree of renal impairment: firstly, the Cockcroft and Gault equation; and secondly the modification of diet in renal disease (MDRD) equation. Details of equations can be found in any current pharmacology textbook. There is also some information on these methods in the BNF (Pharmaceutical Press 2019).

Patients with liver impairment

The liver has a large reserve capacity for the metabolism of drugs; only in cases of advanced liver disease will doses of medications need to be reduced. Patients' liver enzyme profiles may serve as good indicators of underlying liver disease and should be checked if the patient has jaundice, ascites or malnutrition. Drugs requiring extra care in liver disease include warfarin, metformin, benzodiazepines, opioids, NSAIDs, phenytoin and chloramphenicol. Good indicators of reduced hepatic function are an increase in INR and reduced albumin. In these situations, liver-metabolised drug doses may need to be reduced. In some cases, the effects of drugs have been studied in patients with liver disease and specific guidance can be found in the BNF (Pharmaceutical Press 2019) and SmPCs (Datapharm 2019). There are cases where drug effects in liver disease have not previously been studied but it is possible to suggest recommendations based on the drug's pharmacokinetic profile.

Drug choice in complicated liver disease

In patients presenting with liver failure, the risk of complications is high, as these individuals often present with encephalopathy, ascites or visceral bleeding. In this specialist group, doses may need to be reduced, and advice should be sought from the hepatologist to reduce the overall risk and liability.

Hepatic encephalopathy is a disorder that affects the brain and occurs as a result of severe liver disease. It is thought to be due to ammonia being generated by bacteria found in the large bowel, which cannot be adequately removed by the diseased liver. Agents that cause constipation (e.g. opiates and tricyclic antidepressants) should therefore be given with caution or, where appropriate, combined with laxatives. Medications that affect the central nervous system (CNS) should also be given with caution, as they increase the risk (or worsen) encephalopathy. These types of medication include opiates, sedating antihistamines and antipsychotics.

Visceral bleeding can also occur due to impaired coagulopathy, leading to prolonged or excessive bleeding. Coagulopathy is a complication associated with liver disease and hypersplenism. It is caused by chronic portal hypertension and may also lead to conditions such as thrombocytopenia. Drugs that increase the risk of bleeding should therefore be avoided where possible or used with great caution. Drugs that increase the risk of bleeding include NSAIDs (including aspirin), anticoagulants and SSRIs.

Ascites, the accumulation of fluid in the peritoneal cavity, is worsened by high sodium intake and this can lead to further complications in liver disease. Preparations containing sodium chloride as a diluent should therefore be avoided, as should effervescent and soluble drugs due to their high sodium content.

Use of hepatotoxic drugs in liver disease

When using any drug known to be hepatotoxic in patients with liver disease, prescribers should seek advice from a hepatologist to support their clinical judgement. Alternatively, prescribers should consider using another, less hepatotoxic drug to treat the problem. The benefits and risks of prescribing must be carefully weighed up and a decision made as to whether it is more appropriate to delay treatment until the patient's liver function improves. Again, advice from senior and more experienced colleagues may be useful in such situations. This links well with Competency 7 ('Prescribes safely'), which includes statement 7.1: 'prescribes within own scope of practice and recognises the limits of own knowledge and skill'. In addition, Competency 10 ('Prescribes as part of a team') includes statement 10.1, 'acts as part of a multidisciplinary team to ensure that continuity of care across care settings is developed and not compromised' and statement 10.2, 'establishes relationships with other professionals based on understanding, trust and respect for each other's roles in relation to prescribing' (RPS 2016; see Appendix).

Summary

Competency 2 ('Consider the options') includes statement 2.4 'applies understanding of the mode of action and pharmacokinetics of medicines and how these may be altered by e.g. genetics, age, renal impairment and pregnancy'. Accordingly, this chapter has discussed prescribing for neonates and children, older people, pregnant women, breast-feeding women, patients with chronic renal impairment and patients with chronic hepatic impairment. Caution is recommended when prescribing for any of these patient groups. All prescribers, particularly new ones, are encouraged to follow Competency statement 7.1: 'to prescribe within their own scope of practice, recognising the limits of their own knowledge and skill'.

References

Bokhof, B. & Junius-Walker, U. (2016). Reducing polypharmacy from the perspectives of general practitioners and older patients: A synthesis of qualitative studies. *Drugs & Aging.* **33**(4), 249–66.

Bowie, M.W. & Slattum, P.W. (2007). Pharmacodynamics in older adults: a review. *American Journal of Geriatric Pharmacotherapy.* **5**(3), 263–303.

Datapharm (2019). *Electronic Medicine Compendium.* https://www.medicines.org.uk/emc (last accessed 16.5.2019).

Ewen, S., Baumgarten, T. *et al.* (2015). Analyses of drugs stored at home by elderly patients with chronic heart failure. *Clinical Research in Cardiology.* **104**(4), 320–27.

Figueroa, J.J., Basford, J.R. & Low, P.A. (2010). Preventing and treating orthostatic hypotension: As easy as A, B, C. *Cleveland Clinic Journal of Medicine.* **77**(5), 298–306.

García-Poza, P., de Abajo, F.J., *et al.* (2015). Risk of ischemic stroke associated with non-steroidal anti-inflammatory drugs and paracetamol: a population-based case-control study. *Journal of Thrombosis and Haemostasis.* **13**(5), 708–18.

Kaplan, R.C., *et al.* (2001). Risk factors for hospitalized gastrointestinal bleeding among older persons. *Journal of the American Geriatrics Society.* **49**, 126–133.

Klotz, U. (2009). Pharmacokinetics and drug metabolism in the elderly. *Drug Metabolism Reviews.* **41**(2), 67–76.

Laforgia, N., Nuccio, M.M., *et al.* (2014). Off-label and unlicensed drug use among neonatal intensive care units in Southern Italy. *Pediatrics International.* **56**(1), 57–59.

Loke, Y.K. & Singh, S. (2013). Risk of acute urinary retention associated with inhaled anticholinergics in patients with chronic obstructive lung disease: systematic review. *Therapeutic Advances in Drug Safety.* **4**(1), 19–26.

Meador, K.J. & Loring, D.W. (2016). Developmental effects of antiepileptic drugs and the need for improved regulations. *Neurology.* **9**:86(3), 297–306.

Messerli, M., Blozik, E., *et al.* (2016). Impact of a community pharmacist-led medication review on medicines use in patients on polypharmacy – a prospective randomised controlled trial. *BMC Health Services Research.* **23**:16(1), 145.

Medicines and Healthcare products Regulatory Agency (MHRA) (2018). *Guidance; Valproate use by women and girls.* https://www.gov.uk/guidance/valproate-use-by-women-and-girls (last accessed 22.5.2019).

Michielsen, P. & Vandewoude, M. (2010). Liver diseases in the older adult. *Acta Gastro-Enterologica Belgica.* **73**(1), 1–4.

Möller, B., Pruijm, M., *et al.* (2015). Chronic NSAID use and long-term decline of renal function in a prospective rheumatoid arthritis cohort study. *Annals of the Rheumatic Diseases.* **74**(4), 718–23.

National Archives (2012). National Patient Safety Agency. https://webarchive.nationalarchives.gov.uk/20170505131809/ http://www.nrls.npsa.nhs.uk/ (last accessed 22.5.2019).

National Institute for Health and Care Excellence (NICE) (2013). *Falls in older people: assessing risk and prevention.* Clinical Guideline 161. https://www.nice.org.uk/guidance/CG161 (last accessed 22.5.2019).

National Institute for Health and Care Excellence (NICE) (2016). *Epilepsies: diagnosis and management.* Clinical guideline CG137. https://www.nice.org.uk/guidance/cg137 (last accessed 22.5.2019).

National Institute for Health and Care Excellence (NICE) (2017). *Type 2 diabetes: Management.* Clinical Guideline 28. https://www.nice.org.uk/guidance/ng28 (last accessed 22.5.2019).

Obayashi, K., Araki, T., *et al.* (2013). Risk of falling and hypnotic drugs: retrospective study of inpatients. *Drugs in Research and Development.* **13**(2), 159–64.

Office for National Statistics (2018). *Overview of the UK population: November 2018.* https://www.ons.gov.uk/releases/ overviewoftheukpopulationnovember2018 (last accessed 22.5.2019).

Paediatric Formulary Committee (2018). *BNF for Children (2017-2018).* London: Pharmaceutical Press.

Panchaud, A., Weisskopf, E., *et al.* (2014). Pharmacokinetic alterations in pregnancy and use of therapeutic drug monitoring. *Therapie.* **69** (3), 223–34.

Pennell, P.B. (2016). Use of Antiepileptic drugs during pregnancy: Evolving concepts. *Neurotherapeutics.* **13**(4), 811–20.

Pilotto, A. & Franceschi, M. (2003) The risk of upper gastrointestinal bleeding in elderly users of aspirin and other non-steroidal anti-inflammatory drugs: the role of gastro protective drugs. *Aging Clinical and Experimental Research* **15**(6), 494–99.

Pharmaceutical Press (2019). *British National Formulary (BNF)*. London: Pharmaceutical Press.

Royal Pharmaceutical Society (RPS) (2016). *A Competency Framework for All Prescribers*. London: RPS. https://www.rpharms.com/Portals/0/RPS%20document%20library/Open%20access/Professional%20standards/Prescribing%20competency%20framework/prescribing-competency-framework.pdf (last accessed 14.5.2019).

Scheiman, J.M. (2013). The use of proton pump inhibitors in treating and preventing NSAID-induced mucosal damage. *Arthritis Research and Therapy*. **1**(3), S5.

Shah, S., Hall, M., *et al.* (2007). Off-label drug use in hospitalized children. *Archives of Pediatrics and Adolescent Medicine*. **161**(3), 282–90.

Stubbs, B., Denkinger, M.D., *et al.* (2015). What works to prevent falls in older adults dwelling in long term care facilities and hospitals? An umbrella review of meta-analyses of randomised controlled trials. *Maturitas*. **81**(3), 335–42.

Taketomo, C., Hodding, J. & Kraus, D. (2017–2018). *Pediatric & Neonatal Dosage Handbook*. 24 edn. USA: Lex-Comp.

Torstensson, M., Hansen, A.H., *et al.* (2015). Danish register-based study on the association between specific cardiovascular drugs and fragility fractures. *BMJ Open*. **5**(12), e009522.

Toxbase (2019). https://www.toxbase.org/ (last accessed 21.5.2019).

Viazzi, F., Cappadona, F., *et al.* (2016). Chronic kidney disease as a predictor of clinical risk in the elderly. *Journal of Geriatric Cardiology*. **13**(3),199–201.

Victora, C.G. & Bahl, R. (2016). Breastfeeding in the 21st century: epidemiology, mechanisms, and lifelong effect. Lancet Breastfeeding Series Group. *Lancet*. **30**:387(10017), 475–90.

6

Medicines requiring particular care when prescribing

Afthab Hussain

Chapter overview

Whereas the previous chapter concentrated on 'specialist' groups of patients, this chapter concentrates on specific medicines that require particular care when prescribing. Errors can occur and it is the prescriber's responsibility to minimise these by improving their knowledge of individual drugs, gaining more experience in using them, and ensuring they have access to the most up-to-date information about them. In the *Competency Framework for All Prescribers*, the whole of Competency 4 ('Prescribe') covers aspects of safety in prescribing, ensuring that up-to-date information is used (RPS 2016; see Appendix). The drugs and drug groups discussed in this chapter are:

- Anticoagulants
- Insulin
- Opioids
- Antimicrobials
- Oral chemotherapy
- Methotrexate
- Potassium.

Before we consider these specific agents or groups of agents, there is a short section on the potential of certain drugs to cause teratogenicity during pregnancy.

Introduction

From 2002 to 2012, the National Patient Safety Agency (NPSA) collected information regarding medication errors. The information was collected using a national reporting and learning system. The agency's aim was to identify national trends or medication errors and issue national recommendations to reduce the recurrence of such errors. Furthermore, healthcare organisations, including both primary and secondary care providers, have had the responsibility of ensuring that such recommendations are implemented in order to prevent harm to patients.

It's important to bear the following points in mind:

- Although the NPSA website was archived in 2012, many of its reports are still available on the Specialist Pharmacy Services website (see below).
- Alerts issued by NHS England between 2013 and 2016 are still available on the NHS England website (Moore *et al.* 2016).
- All new patient safety alerts (PSAs), issued since 1 April 2016, are available on the NHS Improvement website.
- Many of the NPSA alerts remain available on the Specialist Pharmacy Service (SPS 2019) website.

The following information is taken from the introduction to the SPS website and is printed here with permission of the Specialist Pharmacy Service:

> The Specialist Pharmacy Service pages bring together all the patient safety alerts that relate to medications that were published between 2002 and 2012 by the National Patient Safety Agency (NPSA). Some alerts have, at different points in time, also become Never Events – information can be found on Department of Health website.

Alerts issued between October 2008 and March 2012 can also be found on the Central Alerting System (CAS) website (MHRA 2019). The CAS is a web-based cascading system for issuing patient safety alerts, important public health messages and other safety-critical information and guidance to the NHS and others, including independent providers of health and social care.

The NPSA also supported Signals – Key risks emerging from the review of serious incidents reported by the NHS to its National Reporting and Learning System (NRLS 2019). The issues raised in NPSA Signals are still current. The Specialist Pharmacy Service has created a page on the SPS website of all the medicines-related Signals and SPS Teams have produced resources to support reducing these key risks. A link to the page can be found on https://www.sps.nhs.uk/ then search for 'Signals'.

Where the SPS Medicines Use and Safety Team and/or UK Medicines Information (UKMi 2019) have developed specific resources to support the implementation of an alert, a link is provided via the Word resources for the relevant alert. The alerts are listed by drug or system alphabetically, rather than in chronological order (SPS Medicines Use and Safety Team 2018).

Medication safety

Medication incident reports are reports of errors which actually caused harm, or had the potential to cause harm, involving an error in the process of prescribing, dispensing, preparing, administering, monitoring or providing medicines advice. Of all incidents reported to the NPSA, 90% were associated with low or no harm. The most common reported incidents involved the wrong dose, wrong medicine or often omitted or delayed dispensing of medicines. The NPSA has played a critical role in making sure that the NHS is safer for patients. Competency 7 ('Prescribe safely') includes statement 7.2, 'knows about common types and causes of medication errors and how to prevent, avoid and detect them'. It also includes statement 7.6, 'reports prescribing errors, near misses and critical incidents, and reviews practice to prevent recurrence'. Other parts of the *Competency Framework* include prescribing within own scope of practice, reflecting on your and others' practice, all to the benefit of the patient by improving safety and practice generally (RPS 2016; see Appendix).

Medicines commonly associated with medication errors include anticoagulants, antipsychotics, antiplatelets, insulin, opiates, antibiotics, sedatives, chemotherapeutic agents, methotrexate, infusion fluids and potassium chloride. Due to these agents being associated with medication errors, safety alerts are issued to ensure that particular care is taken when they are prescribed, dispensed and administered.

Drugs with teratogenic and other adverse effects when taken during pregnancy

Warfarin

Warfarin is known to cause teratogenicity and should be avoided in the first trimester. Warfarin is also known to increase the risk of placental and foetal haemorrhage, more commonly during the last trimester. In pregnant women requiring anticoagulation, low molecular weight heparins should be used, such as dalteparin.

Isotretinoin

Isotretinoin is known to cause teratogenicity leading to congenital malformations (Henry *et al.* 2015). It is therefore contraindicated in women of childbearing potential unless all conditions of a pregnancy prevention programme described in the SmPC (Datapharm 2019) are met. If they are met, then the patient must understand and accept the need for effective contraception, without interruption, one month before starting treatment, throughout the duration of treatment and one month after the end of treatment. At least one (and preferably two) complementary forms of contraception, including a barrier method, should be used.

Drugs to treat epilepsy

Anti-epileptic drugs are also teratogenic so it is important to inform women of child-bearing age of the risks to the foetus while taking anti-epileptic medication. Women must be given accurate information and counselling about contraception, conception, pregnancy, caring for children and breast-feeding where the information provided is tailored to the patients' needs (NICE 2016). Patients with epilepsy should be given extensive details on the effect of anti-epileptic drugs and advised on the possible risks of congenital malformations and neurodevelopmental impairment.

In March 2018 the Coordination Group for Mutual Recognition and Decentralised Procedures-human (CMDh) endorsed a strengthened regulatory position on valproate medicines. Valproate must no longer be used in any woman or girl able to have children unless she has a pregnancy prevention programme in place. This is designed to make sure that patients are fully aware of the risks and the need to avoid becoming pregnant while on this medication (MHRA 2018). If unsure, the best course of action as a prescriber is to refer the patient to a consultant neurologist to provide the care. Other anti-epileptics, like carbamazepine and lamotrigine, are known to increase the risk of the foetus developing malformations including cleft palate (Pennell 2016).

Alcohol

Maternal alcohol abuse (both prenatal and postnatal) has been associated with foetal alcohol syndrome, and long-term studies have shown that maternal alcohol abuse can lead to growth deficiency, specific craniofacial dysmorphic features, mental retardation and behavioural changes (Doney & Lucas 2016). Experts are still unsure exactly how much, if any, alcohol is completely safe while pregnant. The safest approach is not to drink at all while pregnant. The Chief Medical Officers for the UK recommend that if pregnant, or planning to become pregnant, the safest approach is not to drink alcohol at all to keep risks to the baby to a minimum (NHS 2017). The latest government and local advice on alcohol use should also be considered.

ACE inhibitors

Recent studies have highlighted an increased overall foetal risk in women who are prescribed angiotensin converting enzyme (ACE) inhibitors during the first trimester. This can lead to a higher risk of cardiovascular and central nervous system malformations, including atrial septal defects, patent ductus arteriosus, hydrocephalus and spina bifida (Li *et al.* 2011). In these patients, medication should be changed to antihypertensives that have better safety profiles. The SmPC can be helpful here.

Antidepressants

Recent studies have associated the use of selective serotonin reuptake inhibitors (SSRIs) with an increase in pre-term birth weights (Eke *et al.* 2016). SSRI use during pregnancy has also been associated with miscarriage, premature birth, cardiac defects, and neurodevelopmental disorders in childhood, specifically autism spectrum disorders (Alwan *et al.* 2016).

However, cessation of antidepressants can lead to a relapse so care must be taken. If the patient has mild depression, stopping treatment may be an option, after discussing the benefits and risks with the patient. If patients have a long history of depression or mental health problems, referral to a consultant in mental health should be considered for close monitoring, support and long-term care. Medical Information Services can also be contacted.

NICE guidance CG 192 (2018) states that:

- Tricyclics such as amitriptyline and imipramine have lower known risks than other antidepressants
- Fluoxetine is the SSRI with the lowest known risk during pregnancy
- Citalopram and fluoxetine are found in relatively high levels in breast milk
- SSRIs taken after week 20 of pregnancy may cause more adverse drug reactions
- Paroxetine in the first trimester may lead to foetal heart defects
- Venlafaxine may be associated with high blood pressure at high doses
- All antidepressants carry the risk of withdrawal or toxicity in neonates.

Corticosteroids

The use of corticosteroids during pregnancy has recently been shown to increase the risk of foetal congenital abnormalities and the use of inhaled corticosteroids has been shown to increase the risk of anal atresia (Garne *et al.* 2016). In the light of this study, care should therefore be taken when prescribing corticosteroids to women before and during pregnancy. Where females have poorly controlled asthma and are considering pregnancy, or if they are already pregnant, they should be referred to a respiratory physician to manage their condition.

Cytotoxic anti-cancer drugs.

Cancer patients should be advised of the risks of anti-cancer drugs for foetal development if they are considering conceiving. Pregnant patients often decide to terminate the pregnancy or delay chemotherapy until after childbirth. Although the cancer is unlikely to affect the child, the chemotherapy agents used to treat the cancer are known to cause congenital defects. Chemotherapy during the first trimester increases the risk of miscarriage and stillbirth and can lead to birth defects. Chemotherapy during the second trimester is considered safer in pregnant women than during the first trimester. Chemotherapy during the second trimester is associated with decreased risk of malformations but the risks of intrauterine growth restriction, low birth weight and stillbirth are still high (Rogers *et al.* 2016). If cancer patients are pregnant, they should be referred urgently to the oncology team for support, counselling and treatment.

Drugs that carry risks for all patients

Apart from specific cases such as pregnancy, the following drugs have been selected to consider in more detail for all patients.

Anticoagulants

The NPSA identified a number of factors that contributed to reported incidents involving anticoagulants. These were primarily due to inadequate competence of healthcare professionals, including those who prescribed for patients on anticoagulant therapy and monitored them. It is therefore imperative that prescribers have the right knowledge, training and competencies before prescribing anticoagulants and that all prescribers work within their scope and limitations of knowledge and skills (Competency 7, statement 7.1). It is also important to remember to reach a shared decision (Competency 3) about treatment, after enough information has been given and understood (RPS 2016; see Appendix).

The NPSA developed six work competencies for anticoagulant therapy. Details of these and other resources can be found on the archived NPSA website (NPSA 2007).

Oral anticoagulants are widely used to treat a number of pathologies, including deep vein thrombosis, pulmonary embolism, arterial thromboembolism and atrial fibrillation (Ferreira & Wipf. 2015). Warfarin is the most common oral anticoagulant prescribed in the UK, and the dose of warfarin given varies from patient to patient. Excessive anticoagulation can result in harm to the patient (through haemorrhage) and under-anticoagulation can potentially result in thrombosis; both are life-threatening conditions (Bauersachs 2016). Warfarin has a narrow therapeutic window and therefore needs to be monitored closely.

The British Committee for Standards in Haematology (BCSH), has produced clear guidelines on oral anticoagulation with warfarin (Keeling *et al.* 2011).

It is common for a patient's INR to become sub-therapeutic or supra-therapeutic. In such cases, the frequency of INR testing should be increased until the INR stabilises again.

Warfarin is known to interact with other drugs and foods and there are also drug–disease interactions. Check in the BNF, Appendix (Pharmaceutical Press 2019).

Cranberry juice can affect warfarin's anticoagulant effects and should be avoided. The BNF (Pharmaceutical Press 2019) explains that, although the interaction is potentially severe, it is anecdotal but still advises avoidance.

Contraindications for warfarin use include:

- Haemorrhagic stroke
- Bleeding disorders
- Pregnancy, due to the teratogenicity of warfarin
- Potential bleeding lesions, e.g. active peptic ulcer, oesophageal varices, aneurysm, proliferative retinopathy or recent surgery.

Cautions in warfarin use include:

- Uncooperative or unreliable patients.
- Patients at risk of recurrent falls are at increased risk of injury and trauma.

Before commencing warfarin, baseline tests must be requested. These include INR, liver function test (LFT), activated partial thromboplastin time (APPT) and total platelets.

Prescribing warfarin for a patient requires knowledge and confidence. Is the patient able to attend for INR monitoring regularly? This can be a problem, especially in those who are frail or confused. Other arrangements may need to be made.

It is important for the prescriber to provide:

- Appropriate and sufficient counselling for the patient regarding the use of anticoagulants
- A patient-orientated booklet, with essential details about warfarin, its potential side effects and how these side effects should be managed and reported
- A card that should be carried at all times by the patient which alerts others that the patient is on warfarin therapy.

Warfarin monitoring

Patients taking warfarin must have regular blood INR tests to allow the dose to be adjusted as necessary. As discussed above, warfarin is known to interact with other drugs, alcohol and diet leading to either an increase or decrease in warfarin's anticoagulant effects.

The prescriber must also keep a record book, in which to record information regarding the patient's dose and INR blood test results. As most patients are initiated on warfarin in secondary care and are then managed in the community, it is critical that all the essential information is recorded in the record book to ensure continuity of care and to reduce the risk of harm to the patient. Take particular note of Competency 4 ('Prescribe'), and in particular statement 4.13, 'communicates information about medicines and what they are being used for when sharing or transferring prescribing responsibilities/ information'.

Unfractionated heparins

Unfractionated heparins have variable anticoagulant and pharmacological effects. Regular blood tests are therefore required to ensure that the desired level of anticoagulation is achieved. The most common test to ensure the required level of anticoagulation is achieved is the activated partial thromboplastin time (APTT) test.

To prevent complications associated with anticoagulation therapies and to reduce risk and harm to patients, it is important that patients are closely monitored and that the dose is adjusted accordingly. It is also important to involve the patient at each step and provide good, clear information, ensuring the patient or their carer is able to understand it. Competency 3 is 'Reach a shared decision' and contains several pointers to ensure that the patient is supported to make an informed decision (RPS 2016; see Appendix).

Low molecular weight heparins (LMWHs)

LMWHs are widely used prophylactically and used to treat venous and arterial thromboembolism. They are prescribed according to the patient's weight and therefore routine monitoring is not required to ensure effective anticoagulation. Common issues seen with LMWHs include: failure of prescribers to weigh patients accurately; failure to identify the clinical need to initiate therapy; and, when therapy is indicated, an inability to calculate the dose accurately.

Patients with renal impairment (RI) will require greater care and consideration, due to potential bioaccumulation. A dose reduction is recommended in patients with severe RI. Limited data on dalteparin and tinzaparin suggest that there is less bioaccumulation with these drugs (Schmid *et al.* 2009). In patients with renal impairment or the elderly, there is an increased risk of bleeding so accurate monitoring is required and these patients will generally require lower doses (Boey & Gallus 2016).

Direct oral anticoagulants (DOACs)

These were formerly known as non-vitamin K oral anticoagulants or novel oral anticoagulants (NOACs). However, DOAC seems to be the appropriate term and it is recommended that it should be embraced by prescribers to describe these newer oral anticoagulants and oral anticoagulants with similar direct mechanisms that haven't yet been released (Kearon *et al.* 2016).

DOACs are a relatively new group of medicines, which affect the production of thrombin. Thrombin enables fibrinogen to be converted to fibrin in the coagulation cascade; inhibiting thrombin therefore prevents the production of a clot (Galanis 2011). DOACs include apixaban, edoxaban and rivaroxaban, which are reversible direct factor Xa inhibitors. (Inhibiting factor Xa in this manner reduces production of thrombin, which increases clotting time and reduces the risk of thrombus formation.) Another DOAC, dabigatran, reversibly inhibits thrombin. These agents are licensed for the prevention of venous thromboembolic events in adults, treatment of deep vein thrombosis or pulmonary embolism (or preventing the recurrence of these events), and prevention of stroke or systemic embolism for patients with non-valvular atrial fibrillation.

The DOACs are a very welcome addition to the anticoagulant class of medicines, as they do not possess similar limitations to warfarin (such as extensive drug and dietary interactions, the necessity for frequent monitoring of INRs and the variable response rate among patients). The DOACs are also advantageous because they display predictable pharmacokinetics, which means that fixed dosing is possible and there is a rapid onset and offset of action in patients. Furthermore, they have predictable pharmacological effects, and therefore do not require frequent testing. However, it is less straightforward to measure a DOAC's activity than it is to measure the Vitamin K antagonists. A DOAC's activity can only be measured through specific clotting assays such as the dilute thrombin time assay (dTT) for dabigatran or a drug-specific anti-Xa chromogenic assay for edoxaban, apixaban and rivaroxaban. These assays are not available within the hospital setting at present (Yip & Chan 2015).

Currently only one specific antidote is licensed to reverse the effects of a DOAC. Idarucizumab, a humanised monoclonal antibody, is licensed for the rapid reversal of dabigatran in emergency situations or in life-threatening or uncontrolled bleeding. Idarucizumab binds to dabigatran with greater affinity than dabigatran binds to thrombin, thus antagonising its anticoagulant effect (Burnett *et al.* 2017).

While the DOACs have fewer drug and dietary interactions than Vitamin K antagonists, they do interact with a variety of substances. These substances include analgesics such as NSAIDs, antidepressants such as St John's Wort, and immunosuppressants such as ciclosporin (Di Minno *et al.* 2017). The SmPCs for each of the DOACs and the latest edition of the BNF are excellent references for complete information on drug and lifestyle interactions with these agents.

Insulin

Insulin is widely used for the management of Type 1 and in many cases Type 2 diabetes mellitus. The NPSA (2011) reported 16,600 cases of medication incidents involving the use of insulin; 24% of these incidents caused significant harm to patients. The causes of patient harm relating to insulin include:

- Inappropriate doses prescribed
- Inappropriate doses administered
- Incorrect type of insulin prescribed or administered
- Delayed or omitted doses
- Inappropriate abbreviations used for units.

Competency 4 ('Prescribe') covers these aspects, particularly statement 4.6, 'accurately completes and routinely checks calculations relevant to prescribing and practical dosing' (RPS 2016; see Appendix).

Insulin prescribing can be confusing, as can its administration. Insulin prescribing errors are known to occur because insulins have similar names – for example, Novorapid and Novomix, or Humulin S and Humulin I. Other insulins can differ in their strength – for example, Humalog, Humalog Mix 25 and Humalog Mix 50. Prescribers therefore need to take care and make sure the correct type and strength of insulin is prescribed. The Department of Health has classified incorrect insulin use as a 'Never Event' (DH 2012).

Prescribers must have the appropriate up-to-date knowledge and training to prescribe insulin in a safe manner – see Competency 4 ('Prescribe') where statement 4.1 is 'prescribes a medicine only with adequate, up to date awareness of its action, indications, dose, contraindications, interactions, cautions and unwanted effects' and Competency 7 ('Prescribe safely') which includes statement 7.1, 'prescribes within own scope of practice and recognises the limits of own knowledge and skill' (RPS 2016; see Appendix). A number of e-learning packages are available online to ensure safe prescribing of insulin; and extensive information on insulin initiation and adjustment is available on the NICE website and many others (NICE 2015, SIGN 2014).

To reduce prescribing errors with insulin, the prescription should include:

● Insulin and the type it is (e.g. Insulin Lispro)
● Brand name (e.g. Lantus)
● The device it is to be used with (e.g. Innolet)
● The dose, stated clearly, and the words for the units need to be written in full.

The NPSA has advised all NHS organisations to issue all patients on insulin with an 'insulin passport'. The aim of the insulin passport is to enable patients to be actively involved in their treatment in order to reduce the risk associated with insulin use. The insulin passport is a valuable document, allowing changes to insulin regimens to be documented. When advising on a patient's diabetes, the prescriber should always refer to the patient's insulin passport before changing insulin levels.

Opioids

The terms opioid and opiate can be confusing. The two are usually differentiated by saying that opiates are alkaloids derived from the opium poppy such as morphine, while opioids such as methadone are synthetic. However, the term opioid is commonly used to refer to the entire family of opiates, including natural, synthetic and semi-synthetic. Opioids are widely used clinically for the treatment of acute or chronic pain. They have also been associated with prescribing errors. Patients can be harmed as a result of inappropriate prescribing and administration of these which is classified as a 'Never Event' (DH 2012). Individuals who have never previously been prescribed opioids may be one group of patients who are more sensitive to their adverse effects.

Before deciding on analgesia, and after a clinical examination of the patient has been conducted, a full medication history is essential. This must include questions on drug allergies and, if considering an opioid, whether the patient has taken opioids in the past (see Chapter 2). If the patient has previously taken opioids, it is important to note the type of medication and the dose taken.

In August 2018, the World Health Organisation published an information sheet on opioid overdose (WHO 2018), which stated:

> Due to their effect on the part of the brain which regulates breathing, opioids in high doses can cause respiratory depression and death. An opioid overdose can be identified by a combination of three signs and symptoms referred to as the 'opioid overdose triad'. The symptoms of the triad are:
>
> ● pinpoint pupils
> ● unconsciousness
> ● respiratory depression.

The BNF provides information on a recommended starting dose, as well as dose conversions from one opioid to another. If prescribing in palliative care, additional information should be sourced from a palliative care formulary and/or local policies and guidelines (Twycross, Wilcock & Howard 2017).

Patients taking opioids will often require dose titration to ensure adequate pain relief. In some cases, an increase in the dose of the opioid will be necessary after ensuring that the new calculated dose is safe for the patient. The dose of opioid should be increased gradually. In palliative care, there may be breakthrough pain between doses of, for example, sustained-release morphine. In this case, an immediate-release dose of morphine, a rescue dose, should be given. The number of such rescue doses can be used to calculate a new higher dose of sustained-release morphine. Increments should not exceed one-third to one-half of the total daily dose every 24 hours. The increase in morphine doses must stop when either the pain is relieved or unacceptable adverse effects occur, after which it is necessary to consider alternative measures (Pharmaceutical Press 2019).

Selecting the wrong product is a common source of error and therefore extensive care in checking is necessary. The Misuse of Drugs Act (2001) places legal requirements on prescribing opioid analgesics that need careful consideration when prescribing.

The WHO information sheet (WHO 2018) recommends the following to help prevent opioid overdose:

> Beyond approaches to reducing drug use in general in the community, specific measures to prevent opioid overdose include:
>
> ● increasing the availability of opioid dependence treatment, including for those dependent on prescription opioids;
> ● reducing irrational or inappropriate opioid prescribing;
> ● monitoring opioid prescribing and dispensing;
> ● limiting inappropriate over-the-counter sales of opioids.
>
> The gap between recommendations and practice is significant. Only half of countries provide access to effective treatment options for opioid dependence and less than 10% of people worldwide in need of such treatment are receiving it.

Antimicrobials

A growing body of evidence suggests that antimicrobials are associated with the highest levels of prescribing errors, potentially affecting both adults and children (Berard *et al.* 2016; Wallace & Paauw 2015). Recent studies have highlighted the risks of inappropriate antimicrobial drug prescribing and how it is contributing to global antibiotic resistance (Holmes *et al.* 2016). Between 2010 and 2013, there was a 6% increase in antibiotic prescribing in England. Furthermore, there was a 4% rise in antibiotic prescribing in general practice and a 12% rise in secondary care prescribing (Public Health England 2017).

In secondary care, antibiotic resistance currently affects 1 in 10 patients, making it difficult to treat them. Furthermore, inappropriate antimicrobial prescribing in hospitals also leads to increased costs and potentially increases the length of the patient's stay. Other common prescribing errors with this type of medication include incorrect dose, incorrect selection of the antibiotic, treatment failure, delayed dosing, omitted doses and adverse drug reactions. Competency 2 ('Consider the options') includes statement 2.10 'understands antimicrobial resistance and the roles of infection prevention control and antimicrobial stewardship measures' (RPS 2016; see Appendix).

One of the reasons for these prescribing errors is often the prescriber's own lack of experience. Inexperienced prescribers generally prescribe broad-spectrum antibiotics, and then short-spectrum ones. Again, incorrect prescribing contributes to the increasing prevalence of antibiotic resistance.

For primary care, Public Health England has introduced guidance called *Managing common infections: guidance for primary care* (Public Health England 2017). This document provides extensive details on the knowledge and principles needed to understand, treat and manage common infections. It also contains links to websites and documents for guidance and further reading.

NHS prescribers and organisations are now signposted to the *TARGET Antibiotic Toolkit* (RCGP 2019) and *Antimicrobial stewardship: Start smart – then focus* toolkits (Public Health England 2011). These toolkits have been developed, with the help of other relevant organisations, to improve antibiotic prescribing in both primary and secondary care.

Once it has been established that there is a bacterial infection, prescribers should follow local prescribing guidelines on antibiotic use. There may be complex patients or some with antibiotic resistance, in which case the results should be discussed with a local clinical microbiologist.

Although it is not always possible or practical, it is good practice to obtain samples from patients before prescribing antibiotics. If available, any microbiology lab report should be taken into consideration and used to inform prescribing decisions. As it says in statement 1.4, the prescriber 'requests and interprets relevant investigations necessary to inform treatment options' (RPS 2016; see Appendix). The number of patients experiencing harm from inappropriate antibiotic prescribing, despite having a documented drug allergy, remains high. Care must therefore be taken at all stages of the prescribing process. Statement 4.12 of Competency 4 is 'makes accurate, legible and contemporaneous records and clinical notes of prescribing decisions' (RPS 2016; see Appendix). In life-threatening situations, such as sepsis, treatment may of course be commenced without a cultures or sensitivities report.

Whatever prescribing decision is taken, it is vital to document all information from the consultation in the patient's medical records. The whole of Competency 4 ('Prescribe') is relevant here (RPS 2016; see Appendix).

Oral chemotherapy

Oral anti-cancer treatments are widely used and administered via primary and secondary care. Anti-cancer agents have been associated with a number of serious safety incidents. Weingart *et al.* (2010), in Boston Massachusetts, identified a number of adverse drug events with oral anti-cancer medication. Some of these were serious or life-threatening, but most were minor near misses, and medical errors with low risk of harm. The most common medication errors involved wrong dose, the wrong drug, the wrong number of days supplied, and missed doses.

A number of issues have been identified with anti-cancer drug prescribing, including:

- Incorrect dose being prescribed
- Incorrect frequency of drugs
- Incorrect duration of prescribed course
- Incorrect route of administration.

Anti-cancer drugs, whether injectable or oral, should only be commenced by a cancer specialist, with a detailed plan of treatment being noted and given to the patient (Felici, Verweij & Sparreboom 2016). The patient should be informed about the treatment at all stages and give their full verbal and written consent for treatment, as in Competency 10 ('Reach a shared decision'). Due to the cytotoxic nature of anti-cancer drugs, regular monitoring is required and the plan for monitoring should also be given to the patient.

The local cancer network can provide prescribers with a range of chemotherapy-related educational resources to read and other material that can be distributed to patients. Competency 10 ('Prescribe as part of a team') encourages prescribers to establish relationships with other professionals (RPS 2016; see Appendix).

Methotrexate

Methotrexate is widely used to treat rheumatoid arthritis, psoriasis, Crohn's disease and autoimmune disorders and is indicated in a number of other conditions (Campbell *et al.* 2016). Methotrexate is a safe and effective medication when taken at the correct dose and monitored correctly. However, when methotrexate is given at an incorrect dose, or not monitored appropriately, this can lead to serious harm and may even be fatal to patients. Primary care clinicians should therefore only accept responsibility for prescribing methotrexate if provided with a shared care agreement from a specialist.

Methotrexate is taken weekly and not on a daily basis to reduce the risk of toxicity (Cairns *et al.* 2016). Patients prescribed methotrexate require routine blood monitoring on therapy initiation, followed by regular repeat tests (including full blood count, liver function tests and renal function tests). Routine blood testing is important and close monitoring is paramount to prevent serious harm to patients. Patients need to be reviewed regularly for signs of methotrexate toxicity or intolerance. Signs of methotrexate toxicity include breathlessness, sore throat, mouth ulcers, bruising, dry persistent cough, vomiting and diarrhoea.

To help facilitate monitoring of patients on methotrexate, all patients are issued with a monitoring booklet. The booklet should give details of the dose being prescribed and the monitoring schedule. Methotrexate works by inhibiting folate metabolism and patients can therefore experience side effects similar to those seen in patients with folate deficiency. Folic acid supplementation is considered in patients who show mucosal or gastrointestinal side effects; folic acid is commonly prescribed alongside methotrexate but not administered on the same day.

Potassium

Potassium is intravenously administered to treat patients with severe or symptomatic hypokalaemia. Potassium solutions are also known sources of potential errors and a number of such incidents have previously been reported to the NPSA. Ampoules of potassium are available as potassium chloride or potassium phosphate; and inappropriate administration of these solutions can be fatal and lead to cardiac arrest and subsequent death. The Department of Health (2012) has also included this as a 'Never Event'.

When prescribing potassium, the concentration of potassium and the rate of infusion need to be considered to ensure that these are safe for the patient. When potassium infusions are being administered, serum potassium, serum electrolytes and blood glucose levels should be monitored at regular intervals. The patient should be examined for signs of pain, confusion, paraesthesia and weakness, vein irritation and extravasation at the site of cannulation. ECGs should also be carried out during infusions, especially at higher concentrations of faster infusions.

Summary

This chapter, using examples of particular drugs, has highlighted commonly reported drug errors and how they can be prevented. For the medicines discussed, there were references to national guidelines that provide information on how each drug should be prescribed. It is strongly recommended that prescribers keep abreast of the developments in the safe and effective use of medicines. The importance of this is highlighted by the emergence of DOACs as a valuable class of medicines in the past decade, the use of which is largely replacing that of Vitamin K antagonists. Likewise, the example of recent safety alerts relating to the use of valproate products in women of child-bearing age illustrates the need to be responsive to new information on the safe use of medicines.

References

Alwan, S., Friedman, J.M. & Chambers, C. (2016). Safety of selective serotonin reuptakeinhibitors in pregnancy: A review of current evidence. *CNS Drugs*. **30**(6), 499–515.

Bauersachs, R. (2016). Non-vitamin K antagonist oral anticoagulants for the prevention of recurrent venous thromboembolism. *Thrombosis Research*. **20**(144), 12–20.

Bérard, C., Cotteret C., *et al*. (2016). Pilot study evaluating the ratio of medication errors related to antimicrobials compared to their consumption. *Archives of Pediatrics and Adolescent Medicine*. **6**, 561–69.

Boey, J.P. & Gallus, A. (2016). Drug treatment of venous thromboembolism in the elderly. *Drugs and Aging*. **33**(7), 475–90.

Burnett, A., Siegal, D. & Crowther, M. (2017). Specific antidotes for bleeding associated with direct oral anticoagulants. *British Medical Journal*. **357**, j2216.

Cairns, R., Brown, J.A., *et al*. (2016). A decade of Australian methotrexate dosing errors. *Medical Journal of Australia*. **204**(10), 384.

Campbell, J.M., Bateman, E., *et al*. (2016). Methotrexate-induced toxicity pharmacogenetics: an umbrella review of systematic reviews and meta-analyses. *Cancer Chemotherapy and Pharmacology*. **78**(1), 27–39.

Department of Health (DH) (2012). *The 'never events' list for 2012/13*. https://www.gov.uk/government/publications/the-never-events-list-for-2012-13 (last accessed 23.5.2019).

Di Minno, A., Frigerio, B., *et al*. (2017). Old and new oral anticoagulants: Food, herbal medicines and drug interactions. *Blood Reviews*. **31**, 193–203.

Doney, R. & Lucas, B.R. (2016). Visual-motor integration, visual perception, and fine motor coordination in a population of children with high levels of Fetal Alcohol Spectrum Disorder. *Research in Developmental Disabilities*. **55**, 346–357.

Eke, A., Saccone, G. & Berghella, V. (2016). Selective serotonin reuptake inhibitor (SSRI) use during pregnancy and risk of preterm birth: a systematic review and meta-analysis. *BJOG An International Journal of Obstetrics and Gynaecology*. **123**(12), 1900–907.

Felici, A., Verweij, J. & Sparreboom, A. (2002). Dosing strategies for anticancer drugs: the good, the bad and body-surface area. *European Journal of Cancer*. **38**(13), 1677–84.

Ferreira, J.L. & Wipf, J.E. (2015). Pharmacologic therapies in anticoagulation. *Medical Clinics of North America*. **100**(4), 695–718.

Galanis, T., Thomson, L., *et al*. (2011). New oral anticoagulants. *Journal of Thrombosis Thrombolysis*. **31**, 310–20.

Garne, E., Vinkel Hansen, A., *et al*. (2016). Risk of congenital anomalies after exposure to asthma medication in the first trimester of pregnancy – a cohort linkage study. *BJOG An International Journal of Obstetrics and Gynaecology*. **123**(10), 1609–618.

Henry, D., Dormuth, C., *et al*. (2016). Occurrence of pregnancy and pregnancy outcomes during isotretinoin therapy. *Canadian Medical Association Journal*. **188**(10), 723–30.

Holmes, A.H., Moore, L.S., *et al*. (2016) Understanding the mechanisms and drivers of antimicrobial resistance. *Lancet*. **387**(10014), 176–87.

Kearon, C, Akl, E.A., *et al*. (2016) Antithrombotic therapy for VTE Disease: CHEST Guideline and Expert Panel Report. *Chest*. **149**(2), 315–52.

Keeling, D., Baglin, T., *et al*. (2011) Guidelines on oral anticoagulation with warfarin. *British Journal of Haematology*. **154**(3), 311–24.

Li, D.K., Yang, C., *et al*. (2011). Maternal exposure to angiotensin converting enzyme inhibitors in the first trimester and risk of malformations in offspring: a retrospective cohort study. *British Medical Journal*. **343**, d5931.

Medicines and Healthcare Products Regulatory Agency (MHRA) (2018). *Guidance: Valproate use by women and girls*. https://www.gov.uk/guidance/valproate-use-by-women-and-girls (last accessed 23.5.2019).

Medicines and Healthcare Products Regulatory Agency (MHRA) (2019). *Central Alerting System*. https://www.cas.mhra.gov.uk/Home.aspx (last accessed 23.5.2019).

Moore, S., Taylor, N., *et al*. (2016). Implementing national patient safety alerts. *Nursing Times*. **112**(11), 12–15.

National Reporting and Learning System (NRLS) (2019). *National Reporting and Learning System. NHS Improvement*. https://improvement.nhs.uk/resources/learning-from-patient-safety-incidents/ (last accessed 20.5.2019).

NHS (2017). *Drinking alcohol while pregnant*. https://www.nhs.uk/conditions/pregnancy-and-baby/alcohol-medicines-drugs-pregnant/ (last accessed 28.5.2019).

NHS England (2014). *An introduction to the NHS England National Patient Safety Alerting System.* https://www.england. nhs.uk/wp-content/uploads/2014/01/npsas-guide.pdf (last accessed 23.5.2019).

NHS Improvement (2016). *Patient safety incident reporting and responding to patient safety alerts.* https://improvement. nhs.uk/news-alerts/patient-safety-incident-reporting-and-responding-patient-safety-alerts/ (last accessed 23.5.2019).

National Institute for Health and Care Excellence (NICE) (2015). *Methotrexate monitoring requirements.* https://cks.nice. org.uk/dmards#!scenario:10 (last accessed 23.5.2019).

National Institute for Health and Care Excellence (NICE) (2018). *Antenatal and postnatal mental health: clinical management and service.* [CG192] https://www.nice.org.uk/guidance/cg192 (last accessed 23.5.2019).

National Patient Safety Agency (NPSA) (2007). *Actions that can make oral anticoagulant therapy safer.* https://www.sps. nhs.uk/articles/npsa-alert-actions-that-can-make-oral-anticoagulant-therapy-safer-2007/ (last accessed 23.5.2019).

National Patient Safety Agency (NPSA) (2008). *Oral anti-cancer medicines: risks of incorrect dosing.* https://www.sps.nhs. uk/articles/npsa-alert-oral-anti-cancer-medicines-risks-of-incorrect-dosing-2008/ (last accessed 23.5.2019).

National Patient Safety Agency (NPSA) (2010). Updated in 2017. *Safer administration of insulin.* https://www.sps.nhs.uk/ articles/npsa-alert-safer-administration-of-insulin-2010/ (last accessed 23.5.2019).

National Patient Safety Agency (NPSA) (2011). *The adult patient's passport to safer use of insulin.* https://www.sps.nhs.uk/ articles/npsa-alert-the-adult-patients-passport-to-safer-use-of-insulin-2011/ (last accessed 23.5.2019).

National Patient Safety Agency (NPSA) (2016). *Patient safety alerts (Including Rapid Response Reports) Safety Alerts from the NPSA and SPS resources to support their implementation.* https://www.sps.nhs.uk/articles/patient-medication-safety-alerts-from-the-npsa-and-sps-resources-to-support-their-implementation/ (last accessed 23.5.2019).

Pennell, P.B. (2016). Use of antiepileptic drugs during pregnancy: Evolving concepts. *Neurotherapeutics.* **13**(4), 811–820.

Pharmaceutical Press (2019). *British National Formulary (BNF).* London: Pharmaceutical Press.

Public Health England (2011). *Antimicrobial stewardship: Start smart – then focus.* https://www.gov.uk/government/ publications/antimicrobial-stewardship-start-smart-then-focus (last accessed 23.5.2019).

Public Health England (2015). *Patient safety alert – addressing antimicrobial resistance through implementation of an antimicrobial stewardship programme.* https://www.england.nhs.uk/wp-content/uploads/2015/08/psa-amr-stewardship-prog.pdf (last accessed 23.5.2019).

Public Health England (2017). *Managing common infections: guidance for primary care.* https://www.gov.uk/government/ consultations/managing-common-infections-guidance-for-primary-care (last accessed 23.5.2019).

Rogers, J.E., Dasari, A., *et al.* (2016). The treatment of colorectal cancer during pregnancy: Cytotoxic chemotherapy and targeted therapy challenges. *The Oncologist.* **21**(5), 563–70.

Royal College of General Practitioners (RCGP) (2019). *TARGET Antibiotic Toolkit.* https://www.rcgp.org.uk/clinical-and-research/resources/toolkits/target-antibiotic-toolkit.aspx (last accessed 23.5.2019).

Royal Pharmaceutical Society (RPS) (2016). *A Competency Framework for All Prescribers.* London: RPS. https://www. rpharms.com/Portals/0/RPS%20document%20library/Open%20access/Professional%20standards/Prescribing%20 competency%20framework/prescribing-competency-framework.pdf (last accessed 14.5.2019).

Schmid, P., Fischer, A.G., *et al.* (2009). Low molecular weight heparin in patients with renal insufficiency. *Swiss Medical Weekly.* **139** (31–32), 438–52.

Scottish Intercollegiate Guidelines Network (SIGN) (2013). *Antithrombotics: indications and management. A national clinical guideline.* https://www.sign.ac.uk/assets/sign129.pdf (last accessed 23.5.2019).

Scottish Intercollegiate Guidelines Network (SIGN) (2014). *Management of diabetes: a national clinical guideline (116).* https://www.sign.ac.uk/assets/sign116.pdf (last accessed 23.5.2019).

Specialist Pharmacy Service (SPS) (2018). *Medicines Use and Safety Team – Annual Report 2017–18.* https://www.sps.nhs. uk/ (last accessed 23.5.2019).

Specialist Pharmacy Service (SPS) (2019). https://www.sps.nhs.uk/ (last accessed 22.5.2019).

Twycross, R., Wilcock, A. & Howard, P. (editors) (2017). *Palliative Care Formulary (2000–2017).* https://www. palliativedrugs.com/assets/pcf5/PCF5_sample_prelims.pdf (last accessed 23.5.2019).

UK Medicines Information (UK/Mi) (2019). http://www.ukmi.nhs.uk/ (last accessed 22.5.2019).

Wallace, J. & Paauw, D.S. (2015). Appropriate prescribing and important drug interactions in older adults. *Medical Clinics of North America.* **99**(2), 295–310.

Weingart, S.N., Toro, J., *et al.* (2010). Medication errors involving oral chemotherapy. *Cancer.* **116**(10), 2455–64.

World Health Organisation (WHO) (2018). *Information sheet on opioid overdose.* https://www.who.int/substance_abuse/information-sheet/en/ (last accessed 23.5.2019).

Yip, S.W. & Chan, Y.C. (2015). Antidotes for patients taking novel oral anticoagulants. *World Journal of Emergency Medicine.* **6**, 31.

Appendix

Section 6.0 The Prescribing Competency Framework Pages 9-14, Royal Pharmaceutical Society A Competency Framework for All Prescribers, July 2016

6.0 THE PRESCRIBING COMPETENCY FRAMEWORK

The competency framework (illustrated below) sets out what good prescribing looks like. There are ten competencies split into two domains. Within each of the ten competency dimensions there are statements which describe the activity or outcomes prescribers should be able to demonstrate.

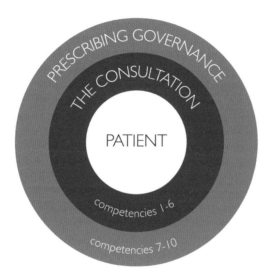

THE CONSULTATION	PRESCRIBING GOVERNANCE
1. Assess the patient	7. Prescribe safely
2. Consider the options	8. Prescribe professionally
3. Reach a shared decision	9. Improve prescribing practice
4. Prescribe	10. Prescribe as part of a team
5. Provide information	
6. Monitor and review	

Figure 1 The prescribing competency framework

THE CONSULTATION (COMPETENCIES 1-6)

1: ASSESS THE PATIENT

1.1 Takes an appropriate medical, social and medication history[1] including allergies and intolerances.

1.2 Undertakes an appropriate clinical assessment.

1.3 Accesses and interprets all available and relevant patient records to ensure knowledge of the patient's management to date.

1.4 Requests and interprets relevant investigations necessary to inform treatment options.

1.5 Makes, confirms or understands, the working or final diagnosis by systematically considering the various possibilities (differential diagnosis).

1.6 Understands the condition(s) being treated, their natural progression and how to assess their severity, deterioration and anticipated response to treatment.

1.7 Reviews adherence to and effectiveness of current medicines.

1.8 Refers to or seeks guidance from another member of the team, a specialist or a prescribing information source when necessary.

2: CONSIDER THE OPTIONS

2.1 Considers both non-pharmacological (including no treatment) and pharmacological approaches to modifying disease and promoting health.

2.2 Considers all pharmacological treatment options including optimising doses as well as stopping treatment (appropriate polypharmacy, de-prescribing).

2.3 Assesses the risks and benefits to the patient of taking or not taking a medicine or treatment.

2.4 Applies understanding of the mode of action and pharmacokinetics of medicines and how these may be altered (e.g. by genetics, age, renal impairment, pregnancy).

2.5 Assesses how co-morbidities, existing medication, allergies, contraindications and quality of life impact on management options.

2.6 Takes into account any relevant patient factors (e.g. ability to swallow, religion) and the potential impact on route of administration and formulation of medicines.

2.7 Identifies, accesses, and uses reliable and validated sources of information and critically evaluates other information.

2.8 Stays up-to-date in own area of practice and applies the principles of evidence-based practice, including clinical and cost-effectiveness.

[1] This includes current and previously prescribed and non-prescribed medicines, on-line medicines, supplements, complementary remedies, illicit drugs and vaccines.

2: CONSIDER THE OPTIONS (CONTINUED)

2.9 Takes into account the wider perspective including the public health issues related to medicines and their use and promoting health.

2.10 Understands antimicrobial resistance and the roles of infection prevention, control and antimicrobial stewardship measures.[2]

3: REACH A SHARED DECISION

3.1 Works with the patient/carer[3] in partnership to make informed choices, agreeing a plan that respects patient preferences including their right to refuse or limit treatment.

3.2 Identifies and respects the patient in relation to diversity, values, beliefs and expectations about their health and treatment with medicines.

3.3 Explains the rationale behind and the potential risks and benefits of management options in a way the patient/carer understands.

3.4 Routinely assesses adherence in a non-judgemental way and understands the different reasons non-adherence can occur (intentional or non-intentional) and how best to support patients/carers.

3.5 Builds a relationship which encourages appropriate prescribing and not the expectation that a prescription will be supplied.

3.6 Explores the patient/carers understanding of a consultation and aims for a satisfactory outcome for the patient/carer and prescriber.

4: PRESCRIBE

4.1 Prescribes a medicine[4] only with adequate, up-to-date awareness of its actions, indications, dose, contraindications, interactions, cautions, and unwanted effects.

4.2 Understands the potential for adverse effects and takes steps to avoid/minimise, recognise and manage them.

4.3 Prescribes within relevant frameworks for medicines use as appropriate (e.g. local formularies, care pathways, protocols and guidelines).

4.4 Prescribes generic medicines where practical and safe for the patient and knows when medicines should be prescribed by branded product.

4.5 Understands and applies relevant national frameworks for medicines use (e.g. NICE, SMC, AWMSG[5] and medicines management/optimisation) to own prescribing practice.

[2] See also Expert Advisory Committee on Antimicrobial Resistance and Healthcare Associated Infections (ARHAI) and Public Health England (PHE) prescribing competencies. https://www.gov.uk/government/publications/antimicrobial-prescribing-and-stewardship-competencies

[3] The term carer is used throughout the prescribing competency framework as an umbrella term that covers care givers, parents and patient advocates or representatives.

[4] For the purpose of the framework medicines can be taken to include all prescribable products.

[5] NICE – National Institute for Health and Clinical Excellence; SMC – Scottish Medicines Consortium; AWMSG – All Wales Medicines Strategy Group

6.0 THE PRESCRIBING COMPETENCY FRAMEWORK

4: PRESCRIBE (CONTINUED)

4.6 Accurately completes and routinely checks calculations relevant to prescribing and practical dosing.

4.7 Considers the potential for misuse of medicines.

4.8 Uses up-to-date information about prescribed medicines (e.g. availability, pack sizes, storage conditions, excipients, costs).

4.9 Electronically generates or writes legible unambiguous and complete prescriptions which meet legal requirements.

4.10 Effectively uses the systems necessary to prescribe medicines (e.g. medicine charts, electronic prescribing, decision support).

4.11 Only prescribes medicines that are unlicensed, 'off-label', or outside standard practice if satisfied that an alternative licensed medicine would not meet the patient's clinical needs[6].

4.12 Makes accurate legible and contemporaneous records and clinical notes of prescribing decisions.

4.13 Communicates information about medicines and what they are being used for when sharing or transferring prescribing responsibilities/ information.

5: PROVIDE INFORMATION

5.1 Checks the patient/carer's understanding of and commitment to the patient's management, monitoring and follow-up.

5.2 Gives the patient/carer clear, understandable and accessible information about their medicines (e.g. what it is for, how to use it, possible unwanted effects and how to report them, expected duration of treatment).

5.3 Guides patients/carers on how to identify reliable sources of information about their medicines and treatments.

5.4 Ensures that the patient/carer knows what to do if there are any concerns about the management of their condition, if the condition deteriorates or if there is no improvement in a specific time frame.

5.5 When possible, encourages and supports patients/carers to take responsibility for their medicines and self-manage their conditions.

[6] At the time of publication only doctors, dentists, nurses and pharmacists are able to independently prescribe unlicensed medicines

6: MONITOR AND REVIEW

6.1 Establishes and maintains a plan for reviewing the patient's treatment.

6.2 Ensures that the effectiveness of treatment and potential unwanted effects are monitored.

6.3 Detects and reports suspected adverse drug reactions using appropriate reporting systems.

6.4 Adapts the management plan in response to on-going monitoring and review of the patient's condition and preferences.

PRECRIBING GOVERNANCE (COMPETENCIES 7-10)

7: PRESCRIBE SAFELY

7.1 Prescribes within own scope of practice and recognises the limits of own knowledge and skill.

7.2 Knows about common types and causes of medication errors and how to prevent, avoid and detect them.

7.3 Identifies the potential risks associated with prescribing via remote media (telephone, email or through a third party) and takes steps to minimise them.

7.4 Minimises risks to patients by using or developing processes that support safe prescribing particularly in areas of high risk (e.g. transfer of information about medicines, prescribing of repeat medicines).

7.5 Keeps up to date with emerging safety concerns related to prescribing.

7.6 Reports prescribing errors, near misses and critical incidents, and reviews practice to prevent recurrence.

8: PRESCRIBE PROFESSIONALLY

8.1 Ensures confidence and competence to prescribe are maintained.

8.2 Accepts personal responsibility for prescribing and understands the legal and ethical implications.

8.3 Knows and works within legal and regulatory frameworks affecting prescribing practice (e.g. controlled drugs, prescribing of unlicensed/off label medicines, regulators guidance, supplementary prescribing).

8.4 Makes prescribing decisions based on the needs of patients and not the prescriber's personal considerations.

8.5 Recognises and deals with factors that might unduly influence prescribing (e.g. pharmaceutical industry, media, patient, colleagues).

8.6 Works within the NHS/organisational/regulatory and other codes of conduct when interacting with the pharmaceutical industry.

9: IMPROVE PRESCRIBING PRACTICE

9.1 Reflects on own and others prescribing practice, and acts upon feedback and discussion.

9.2 Acts upon colleagues' inappropriate or unsafe prescribing practice using appropriate mechanisms.

9.3 Understands and uses available tools to improve prescribing
(e.g. patient and peer review feedback, prescribing data analysis and audit).

10: PRESCRIBE AS PART OF A TEAM

10.1 Acts as part of a multidisciplinary team to ensure that continuity of care across care settings is developed and not compromised.

10.2 Establishes relationships with other professionals based on understanding, trust and respect for each other's roles in relation to prescribing.

10.3 Negotiates the appropriate level of support and supervision for role as a prescriber.

10.4 Understands and uses available tools to improve prescribing
(e.g. patient and peer review feedback, prescribing data analysis and audit).

Index